Veterans' Health Insurance Coverage Under the Affordable Care Act and Implications of Repeal for the Department of Veterans Affairs

Michael Dworsky, Carrie M. Farmer, Mimi Shen

Sponsored by the Robert Wood Johnson Foundation and the New York State Health Foundation

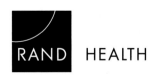

RAND HEALTH

For more information on this publication, visit www.rand.org/t/rr1955

Library of Congress Cataloging-in-Publication Data is available for this publication.

ISBN: 978-0-8330-9891-7

Published by the RAND Corporation, Santa Monica, Calif.

© Copyright 2017 RAND Corporation

RAND® is a registered trademark.

Support RAND
Make a tax-deductible charitable contribution at
www.rand.org/giving/contribute

www.rand.org

Preface

The Affordable Care Act (ACA) has led to historic reductions in the proportion of adults without health insurance, but the law has been controversial, and Republican members of Congress have opposed the law since its passage. After the 2016 presidential election, President Donald Trump and Congress affirmed that repeal of the ACA would be a top legislative priority. The House of Representatives passed the American Health Care Act (AHCA) on May 4, 2017, and the Senate has been considering similar legislation to repeal significant aspects of the ACA and introduce new health reforms.

Repealing the ACA could have a significant effect on U.S. military veterans' health insurance coverage and use of health care from the U.S. Department of Veterans Affairs (VA). Besides providing a new coverage option to veterans who are not enrolled in VA, the ACA also had the potential to affect health care use among VA patients. Although prior research has shown that the number of uninsured veterans fell after the ACA took effect, the implications of ACA repeal for veterans and, especially, for VA have received less attention.

This report presents the findings of a study sponsored by the Robert Wood Johnson Foundation and the New York State Health Foundation. This study had two goals: to describe the ACA's effects on nonelderly veterans' insurance coverage and demand for VA health care and to assess the coverage and VA utilization changes that could result from repealing the ACA. This report uses data from the American Community Survey to measure changes in insurance coverage for nonelderly veterans (under age 65) after the ACA was implemented. Specific areas of emphasis included changes in non-VA insurance coverage among those with VA coverage, the effects of state Medicaid expansion decisions, and effects on subgroups of veterans distinguished by eligibility for VA care and geographic proximity to VA facilities. To quantify the effects of ACA repeal, this study combined VA population estimates, data from federal household surveys, and microsimulation output from RAND's COMPARE model to analyze how coverage changes similar to those anticipated under the AHCA would affect veterans' use of health care from VA and other sources.

At the time this report was finalized (August 2017), the future of efforts to roll back the ACA's coverage expansions remained unclear, and enactment of the AHCA appeared unlikely. The ACA remains controversial, however, and policy changes included in the AHCA could well reemerge in future legislation. The estimates reported here will thus provide a useful starting point for understanding how veterans would fare under future proposals involving similar changes to the individual market or major reductions in federal Medicaid contributions. This report may be of interest to federal and state policymakers. The analysis of VA use presented here may be relevant for VA policy planning. In the event that legislation similar to the AHCA becomes law, community groups concerned with ensuring that veterans have continued access to health care may also find these estimates of use.

Support for this research was provided by the Robert Wood Johnson Foundation and the New York State Health Foundation. The views expressed here do not necessarily reflect the views of the Robert Wood Johnson Foundation. The mission of the New York State Health Foundation is to expand health insurance coverage, increase access to high-quality health care services, and improve public and community health. The views presented here are those of the authors and not necessarily those of the New York State Health Foundation or its directors, officers, and staff.

This research was conducted by RAND Health, a division of the RAND Corporation. Additional information about RAND Health can be found at www.rand.org/health.

Contents

Figures and Tables

Figures

Tables

Summary

The Affordable Care Act (ACA) considerably changed the U.S. health insurance landscape. Among other provisions, the ACA required all adults to obtain health insurance and facilitated this by allowing states to expand Medicaid eligibility to low-income adults, requiring large employers to offer health insurance as a benefit, creating a regulated Marketplace for nongroup health insurance, and providing premium subsidies to help low- and moderate-income adults afford Marketplace coverage. The ACA has led to historic reductions in the proportion of adults without health insurance, but the law has been controversial, and Republican members of Congress have opposed the law since its passage. After the 2016 presidential election, President Donald Trump and Congress affirmed that repeal of the ACA would be a top legislative priority, and the U.S. House of Representatives passed the American Health Care Act (AHCA) on May 4, 2017. The Better Care Reconciliation Act, an amended version of the AHCA, failed to pass the Senate in July 2017, and the path forward for ACA repeal is currently uncertain: President Trump and some congressional Republicans have continued to express strong interest in repealing and replacing the ACA, while other congressional Republicans have voiced interest in improving the law on a bipartisan basis. Debate over the future of the ACA and federal health care reform thus appears likely to continue.

Repealing the ACA could have a significant effect on U.S. military veterans' health insurance coverage and use of health care from the U.S. Department of Veterans Affairs (VA). Veterans are less likely to be uninsured than demographically similar nonveterans, in large part because many have access to VA health care. However, only about one-half of nonelderly veterans (under age 65) are eligible for VA care, and not all who are eligible choose to enroll: Almost one in ten nonelderly veterans lacked any insurance or VA coverage in 2013. Insurance coverage obtained as a result of the ACA had the potential to increase access to care for veterans who are ineligible for or not enrolled in VA.

Besides providing a new coverage option to veterans who are not enrolled in VA, the ACA also had the potential to affect health care use among VA patients. Most VA patients consume a mix of health care from VA and non-VA sources. By making non-VA insurance more widely available to VA enrollees, the ACA may have led some veterans to substitute non-VA care for VA care, perhaps reducing demands on the VA system. Repealing the ACA or introducing additional health system reforms could change both veterans' rates of insurance coverage and, for those veterans using VA care, their patterns of VA health care use.

This study had two goals: to describe the ACA's effects on nonelderly veterans' insurance coverage and demand for VA health care and to assess the coverage and VA utilization changes that could result from repealing the ACA. We used nationally representative data from the American Community Survey (ACS) to estimate changes following implementation of the ACA in veterans' insurance status and VA coverage and data from the Medical Expenditure Panel Survey to model how use of VA health care is affected by changes in non-VA insurance coverage. For our analyses of the potential impact of repeal, we used our estimates of post-ACA coverage changes to quantify how demand for VA care would have differed if the coverage changes that followed the ACA had been reversed. We also drew on microsimulation results from RAND's Comprehensive Assessment of Reform Efforts (COMPARE) model to develop scenarios based on the coverage changes that would result from the AHCA in two future years: 2020 and 2026. For all analyses, we produced both nationwide estimates and state-level estimates for states with large populations of nonelderly veterans.

Insurance Coverage for Nonelderly Veterans Increased After the ACA

In our analysis of the 2013–2015 ACS, we used statistical models to adjust for the changing demographics of the nonelderly veteran population. Figures reported in this summary are adjusted estimates for the 2015 nonelderly veteran population unless otherwise noted.

- In 2013, prior to the major coverage expansions under the ACA, nearly one in ten nonelderly veterans (9.1 percent) were uninsured, lacking access to both VA coverage and non-VA health insurance.
- Uninsurance among nonelderly veterans fell by 36 percent (3.3 percentage points) after implementation of the ACA, from 9.1 percent in 2013 to 5.8 percent in 2015.
- The drop in uninsurance among nonelderly veterans can be attributed to increased Medicaid enrollment due to Medicaid expansion and increased private coverage, including direct-purchase coverage obtained through the ACA Marketplace.
- Nationwide enrollment in Medicaid increased by 2.6 percentage points for nonelderly veterans. Veterans who became newly eligible due to Medicaid expansion experienced the largest increases in Medicaid coverage and the largest reductions in uninsurance. However, Medicaid coverage rose and uninsurance fell for previously Medicaid-eligible veterans in both expansion and nonexpansion states.
- Among low-income nonelderly veterans, Medicaid expansion increased enrollment in Medicaid by 8.4 percentage points relative to similar veterans in nonexpansion states.
- Medicaid expansion led to larger coverage increases for low-income veterans living far from VA facilities, suggesting that Medicaid expansion may have provided a valuable new coverage option for veterans facing barriers to accessing VA.
- The largest reductions in the proportion of veterans without insurance were concentrated in Medicaid expansion states, particularly Oregon, Arkansas, Nevada, Kentucky, and Washington.
- VA coverage among nonelderly veterans increased by 1.3 percentage points after the ACA, but this continued a long-standing trend of increased VA enrollment that preceded the ACA. It is unclear what effect the ACA had on VA enrollment over and above other factors.

VA-Enrolled Veterans Who Gained Insurance After the ACA Likely Reduced Their Use of VA Health Care

We examined the relationship between having non-VA health insurance and both total and VA health care use. VA patients with non-VA health insurance have lower VA demand for office-based visits and prescription drugs, after accounting for differences in demographics, income, and health status between veterans with and without non-VA insurance. To understand how gains in insurance coverage following ACA implementation likely affected VA patients' use of VA health care, we combined those estimates with findings from the research literature and modeled how use of VA health care in 2015 would have changed if veterans' insurance coverage had resembled the lower levels observed in 2013.

- After the ACA, fewer nonelderly veterans were enrolled in VA without another source of coverage. VA-Medicaid dual enrollment increased by 2.7 percentage points between 2013 and 2015. Increases in dual VA-Medicaid coverage were especially pronounced for disabled and low-income VA enrollees.
- By increasing non-VA health insurance coverage for VA patients, the ACA likely led to a decrease in demand for VA care. We estimate that, if the gains in insurance coverage that occurred between 2013 and 2015 had not occurred, nonelderly veterans would have used about 1 percent more VA health care in 2015: 125,000 more office visits, 1,500 more inpatient surgeries, and 375,000 more prescriptions.

Our estimates of changes in VA health care use do not account for concurrent VA policy changes, which may have had an independent effect on nonelderly veterans' use of VA health care.

Repealing the ACA Would Increase the Number of Uninsured Nonelderly Veterans and Slightly Increase Demand for VA Health Care

We then assessed how changes in coverage similar to those forecast under the AHCA could affect veterans' use of VA and total health care by modeling the effects that such coverage changes would have had on demand for care in 2015. We also used population estimates from VA and information on state Medicaid expansion status to produce state-specific estimates of the AHCA's potential impact on VA demand in all 50 states and the District of Columbia.

- Simply reversing the coverage gains that occurred after ACA implementation would increase the proportion of nonelderly veterans without insurance from 5.8 percent to 9.1 percent, a 3.3-percentage-point increase.
- Efforts to repeal and replace the ACA with health reforms that substantially reduce the federal government's role in financing Medicaid could potentially result in lower rates of insurance coverage for low-income veterans otherwise unaffected by the ACA's coverage expansions.
- If the United States were to adopt health care reforms similar to those proposed in the AHCA, a greater proportion of nonelderly veterans would lose insurance than gained coverage after the ACA took effect:
  - If the 2020 AHCA provisions had been in place in 2015, 9.6 percent of nonelderly veterans would have been uninsured. Increased insurance coverage for younger, healthier, higher-income nonelderly veterans would have been offset by decreases in insurance coverage for other groups of nonelderly veterans.
  - If the 2026 AHCA provisions had been in place in 2015, 10.4 percent of nonelderly veterans would have been uninsured. Insurance coverage would have been lower for all groups of nonelderly veterans.

- Losses in insurance coverage resulting from the AHCA would lead nonelderly veterans to cut back on overall use of health care while increasing their use of VA care.

  - VA patients would have received less health care overall (1.7 percent fewer office-based visits and 1.7 percent fewer prescriptions) but more VA health care (2.3 percent more VA office-based visits and 3.2 percent more VA prescriptions) under the 2026 provisions of the AHCA.
  - Increased VA use by nonelderly veterans would have translated into an estimated annual increase of 245,000 VA visits and 910,000 VA prescriptions, or 1 percent and 1.4 percent of total VA use in 2015.

- Medicaid expansion states with higher proportions of low-income and nonelderly veterans would have experienced the largest increases in VA demand as a result of the AHCA, with Arkansas, Kentucky, and Louisiana experiencing the largest increases in VA demand relative to total VA use. Conversely, increases in VA use would be smallest for nonexpansion states with older veteran populations, such as Nebraska, Wisconsin, and Wyoming.

We caution readers that our analyses of the impact of repeal should not be considered forecasts of future VA demand. The nonelderly veteran population is decreasing in size and changing in composition, which will affect demand for VA care in the future. We also do not account for concurrent policy changes that will affect VA demand, such as those aimed at increasing access to care. Instead, our estimates represent the impact that coverage changes similar to those predicted under the AHCA would have had on health care use by the 2015 veteran population.

Our analysis found that the AHCA's effect on veterans' use of VA care would be larger than the effect of simply undoing the coverage gains that occurred after the ACA went into effect. This is because the insurance market changes and reductions in Medicaid spending proposed under the AHCA would primarily affect older, lower-income, and less-healthy nonelderly veterans. These are the same populations of veterans who tend to use the most health care from VA, meaning that the distribution of coverage changes across population groups under the AHCA would tend to magnify the potential increase in VA use that would result from the AHCA's implementation. Legislative proposals that lead to similar patterns of coverage changes across groups of veterans would likely have a similar impact on VA demand.

Some potentially important provisions of the AHCA were not incorporated into the microsimulation estimates we used to analyze ACA repeal. The AHCA and similar legislation would also weaken key consumer protections established under the ACA, such as restrictions that prevent medical underwriting (the practice of using information about a customer's health status in deciding whether to sell insurance and what premium to charge). Such changes may affect the insurability of the estimated 34 percent of nonelderly veterans with preexisting health conditions—and may affect the insurability of a substantially higher share of veterans eligible for VA health care.

At the time this report was finalized (August 2017), an amended version of the AHCA had failed to pass the Senate. The short-term future of efforts to roll back the ACA's coverage expansions thus remains unclear. Even so, the findings of our analysis provide valuable information on the interaction between veterans' access to non-VA health insurance and their use of VA care. While enactment of the AHCA might currently appear unlikely, policy changes included in the AHCA could well reemerge in future legislation. The estimates reported here will thus provide a useful starting point for understanding how veterans would fare under future proposals involving similar changes to the individual market or major reductions in federal Medicaid contributions.

Policymakers considering reforms that would reduce veterans' access to non-VA insurance coverage should be careful to account for potential spillover effects on VA demand. In the event that a law similar to the AHCA is enacted, our findings that older, low-income, and less-healthy veterans would experience the largest changes in coverage may be of interest to federal and state policymakers and VA, as well as community groups concerned with ensuring that veterans have continued access to health care and adequate financial protection from the risk of catastrophic medical expenses.

Acknowledgments

We gratefully acknowledge funding support for this research from the New York State Health Foundation and the Robert Wood Johnson Foundation. We appreciate the comments provided by our reviewers, Jonah Czerwinski and Susan Hosek. Their constructive critiques were addressed as part of RAND's rigorous quality assurance process to improve the quality of this report. We are grateful to several RAND researchers who shared their work with us: Jodi Liu and Christine Eibner for estimates from the COMPARE model, Phillip Armour for his algorithm to estimate veterans' VA enrollment priority groups using ACS data, Joshua Mendelsohn for estimates of veterans' distance to VA health care facilities, and Ernesto Amaral and Kandice Kapinos for their ACS and MEPS analysis code. We thank Anthony Damico and his co-authors at the Kaiser Family Foundation for sharing analysis code to identify preexisting conditions using NHIS data. Finally, we thank Nora Spiering for her editorial assistance and Laura Pavlock-Albright for her administrative support as we prepared this report.

Abbreviations

ACA	Affordable Care Act
ACS	American Community Survey
AHCA	American Health Care Act
BCRA	Better Care Reconciliation Act
CBO	Congressional Budget Office
COMPARE	Comprehensive Assessment of Reform Efforts
CPI-M	Medical Consumer Price Index
ESI	employer-sponsored insurance
FPL	federal poverty level
IHS	Indian Health Service
IPUMS	Integrated Public Use Microdata Series
MEPS	Medical Expenditure Panel Survey
NHIS	National Health Interview Survey
PUMA	Public Use Microdata Area
VA	U.S. Department of Veterans Affairs
VAMC	VA Medical Center

1. Background

The Affordable Care Act (ACA) introduced dramatic changes to the U.S. health insurance and health care delivery landscape by aiming to increase health insurance rates through several channels. The ACA expanded insurance coverage by expanding Medicaid eligibility, creating insurance Marketplaces operated by the states or the federal government, providing premium tax credits for low-income individuals, instituting mandates for most individuals to obtain insurance coverage and for businesses with 50 or more workers to offer coverage, and initiating numerous other reforms. By March 2017, approximately 20 million people were newly enrolled in health insurance, including 12.2 million enrolled in Marketplace plans (Centers for Medicare & Medicaid Services, 2017a) and 17.7 million newly enrolled in Medicaid and the Children's Health Insurance Program (Centers for Medicare & Medicaid Services, 2017b). The ACA has faced considerable political opposition since its enactment, however. Since the November 2016 U.S. presidential election, President Donald Trump and Congress have been engaged in efforts to repeal the ACA and enact new health system reforms.

While the ACA did not directly affect U.S. military veterans' eligibility to enroll in or receive health care as a benefit through the U.S. Department of Veterans Affairs (VA), the new insurance coverage options created by the ACA had the potential to affect nonelderly (under age 65) veterans' insurance status and use of VA care through several channels. Most nonelderly veterans are not enrolled in VA health care—many are not eligible, and among those who are eligible, not all decide to enroll in VA health care. Nonelderly veterans who are not enrolled in VA must obtain health insurance and health care from non-VA sources. Insurance coverage obtained as a result of the ACA had the potential to increase access to care for veterans who are ineligible for or not enrolled in VA. For those veterans who are enrolled in VA, most consume a mix of health care from VA and non-VA sources; two-thirds of nonelderly VA enrollees are covered by public or private insurance outside VA (Gasper et al., 2015). By making non-VA insurance available to VA enrollees, the ACA might also have changed nonelderly veterans' patterns of VA health care use by making other sources of care more accessible.

As debate continues over the future of the ACA and the federal government's role in providing health insurance, there are several reasons to consider the law's impact on veterans' insurance status and patterns of health care use. Veterans tend to have greater health care needs than the nonveteran population, and veterans' access to care is a matter of keen public concern (Eibner et al., 2015). While discussion of veterans' access to care often centers on the VA system, non-VA health insurance can expand veterans' options for seeking care and improve access outside the VA system; such options may be particularly important for those who prefer non-VA doctors or who face geographic barriers to using VA care. For veterans who are ineligible for VA care, non-VA health insurance coverage is likely critical for access to health care. There is also potential for changes in the health insurance landscape to have budgetary impacts on the VA system insofar as veterans' VA enrollment decisions and use of VA care are responsive to non-VA insurance.

To understand the potential impact of ACA repeal on nonelderly veterans' health care use, we first examined empirically how the ACA affected veterans' health insurance coverage and use of VA health care and then estimated how repealing the law might affect these outcomes. For our repeal analysis, we estimated both the impact of reversing the coverage gains from the ACA and the impact of the American Health Care Act (AHCA), legislation to repeal and replace the ACA passed by the House of Representatives in May 2017. In particular, our analysis of the AHCA is based on a RAND analysis of the AHCA as amended March 20, 2017. Key provisions modeled include changes to premium tax credits, elimination of cost-sharing reductions, repeal of the individual and employer mandates, elimination of enhanced federal funding for the ACA Medicaid expansion, and conversion of federal Medicaid funding to a capped allocation. Many of these provisions were retained in some form in the Better Care Reconciliation Act (BCRA), an amended version of the AHCA that was introduced in the Senate. The AHCA and BCRA also included other provisions that we did not analyze quantitatively. Where possible, we discuss how these other changes, such as broadening state waiver authority and loosening regulations on benefit design, might affect veterans and VA.

ACA Repeal Could Affect Nonelderly Veterans' Insurance Coverage and Use of VA Health Care

Of the 21 million veterans in the United States, only those under age 65 (nonelderly veterans) were directly affected by the coverage provisions of the ACA. Nonelderly veterans constitute half (51 percent) of the noninstitutionalized U.S. veteran population; in 2015, there were 10.8 million nonelderly, noninstitutionalized U.S. veterans (Table 1.1). Throughout this report, we use *nonelderly veterans* to refer to the nonelderly, noninstitutionalized veteran population. Veterans age 65 or older are generally covered by Medicare, eligibility for which was not affected by the ACA; therefore, in this study, we focused on changes in coverage and VA use for the nonelderly veteran population.

Table 1.1. Nonelderly U.S. Veterans (2015)

Characteristic	Percentage of Nonelderly U.S. Veterans (2015) (10.8 million total)
Female	13.8%
Age < 50	48.4%
White, non-Hispanic	70.0%
Service era	
Post-9/11	32.8%
Gulf War	24.7%
Between Vietnam and Gulf War	29.0%
Vietnam	13.5%
Income < 200% FPL	22.2%

SOURCES: Authors' calculations, 2015 Integrated Public Use Microdata Series (IPUMS) American Community Survey (ACS) (Ruggles et al., 2015). Total number of nonelderly, noninstitutionalized veterans from VetPop2016 (VA National Center for Veterans Analysis and Statistics, 2017) and the ACS.
NOTE: FPL = federal poverty level.

As noted above, not all nonelderly veterans enrolled in VA health care: In 2016, the VA Survey of Veteran Enrollees' Health and Use of Health Care reported that 38 percent of nonelderly veterans were enrolled in VA (Huang et al., 2017). To enroll, veterans must submit an application and undergo an eligibility determination. Eligible veterans generally must have served at least two years (unless they incurred a disability early in their service) and have an other-than-dishonorable discharge, service during wartime or in combat, a health care condition connected to military service, lower income, or another qualifying characteristic.

Eligible veterans are sorted into enrollment priority groups based on the severity of their service-connected health care conditions, incomes, and other factors. While enrolled veterans do not pay enrollment fees, monthly premiums, or deductibles, veterans in lower-priority groups are required to pay co-pays for some or all the care they receive from VA. We used an algorithm previously developed by RAND to categorize nonelderly veteran ACS respondents into VA enrollment priority groups, based on income, service era, service-connected

VA ENROLLMENT PRIORITY GROUPS

- VA health care enrollment is determined by assigning eligible veterans to enrollment "priority groups." Higher-priority groups include veterans with disabling service-connected disabilities, low incomes, or special circumstances (e.g., Purple Heart recipients). Lower-priority groups include veterans with nondisabling service-connected conditions and higher incomes.
- Veterans in low-priority groups face modest co-pays for VA care ($15 for a primary care visit and $50 for a specialty care visit). This could make non-VA care or dual enrollment somewhat more attractive to low-priority group veterans.
- Compared with high-priority group veterans, low-priority group veterans may have better functional status and greater access to non-VA health insurance.
- We used an algorithm developed for a previous study to assign nonelderly veterans in the ACS to a priority group (Eibner et al., 2015).

disability rating, and functional status.[1] Since we did not have access to VA data, this was by definition an imperfect estimate of nonelderly veterans' eligibility for VA health care and priority group assignment. The algorithm uses a series of actuarial adjustments to ensure that counts of veteran enrollees match administrative totals reported by VA (Appendix A). Differences between priority groups may be underestimated if veterans are misclassified. Using this algorithm, we estimated that 56.8 percent of nonelderly veterans were eligible for enrollment in VA health care in 2015.

Among veterans who are enrolled in VA health care, most use VA to meet only a portion of their health care needs, receiving the remainder of their health care from another source. Most veterans under age 65 have health insurance coverage from a source other than VA (e.g., employer-sponsored insurance, other private insurance, Medicaid, or TRICARE). On average, veterans who use VA health care receive about 30 percent of all of their health care from VA (Eibner et al., 2015). About 40 percent of enrolled veterans use no VA health care during the year (Huang et al., 2017). Veterans choose to use VA health care versus other sources of care for a variety of reasons, including accessibility of care, perceived quality of care, and costs.

While the ACA did not affect veterans' eligibility for VA health care, the law could have affected eligible veterans' VA enrollment and use of VA care through several channels. Expanded availability of non-VA insurance options might affect eligible veterans' decisions about whether to enroll in VA and, if already enrolled, how much VA health care to use. For example, VA-enrolled veterans who gained Medicaid coverage as a result of Medicaid expansion under the ACA may seek care from a non-VA provider and therefore reduce the amount of care they received from VA. Similarly, some eligible veterans who would otherwise have enrolled in VA might choose not to enroll. These factors may tend to reduce demand for VA care. However, the ACA's individual mandate may also have pushed some eligible but unenrolled veterans to enroll to avoid the individual mandate's tax penalty.

State Characteristics and Differences in the Composition of the Nonelderly Veteran Population Mean That the Impact of ACA Repeal Will Vary by State

The age structure of the veteran population differs widely across states, with the nonelderly proportion ranging from an estimated 45 percent in New Jersey to 72 percent in Alaska as of 2015 (U.S. Department of Veterans Affairs National Center for Veterans Analysis and Statistics, 2016). In general, the share of nonelderly veterans as a proportion of the total state veteran population is higher in western and southern states and lower in northeastern states; within the nonelderly veteran population, there are also differences in the geographic distribution of veterans by age and service era (Eibner et al., 2015). The effect of ACA repeal on nonelderly veterans will vary with state characteristics, such as state decisions to expand Medicaid, while the degree to which these changes have a meaningful impact on demand for VA care will vary with the size of the nonelderly veteran population. We note state differences throughout this report; complete tables of our results by state are available in Appendix B.

---

[1] See Appendix A. Appendixes A and B are available for download at www.rand.org/t/RR1955.

ACA Repeal and Replace Plans Are Evolving, but Common Themes Are Evident

The U.S. House of Representatives passed the AHCA, which would repeal parts of the ACA, on May 4, 2017. At the time of this writing, the U.S. Senate had failed to pass a series of ACA repeal bills and was considering new legislative proposals. While the future of ACA repeal is uncertain, it is likely that future legislation will retain many of the key provisions in the AHCA affecting Americans' access to health insurance. In particular, the AHCA would decouple the value of premium tax credits provided under the ACA from the price of insurance, replace the ACA's individual-coverage mandate with a penalty for lapses in continuous coverage, phase out the ACA's Medicaid expansion, and convert Medicaid from an open-ended entitlement to a block grant or per capita allocation.

In addition to reductions in federal spending on premium tax credits and Medicaid, the AHCA would dramatically expand the ability of states to obtain waivers for many of the insurance regulations and consumer protections included under the ACA. Waivers could allow the sale of insurance plans that would violate the requirements under current law that non-grandfathered insurance policies in the individual and small group markets cover a specified set of essential health benefits.

There have been estimates of the effect of repealing the ACA on the number and proportion of individuals covered by health insurance (Congressional Budget Office [CBO], 2017a; Saltzman and Eibner, 2016), as well as estimates of the specific effects of the AHCA (Eibner, Liu, and Nowak, 2017; CBO, 2017a) and similar legislation introduced in the Senate (CBO, 2017b). These studies predict substantial increases in the number of uninsured adults relative to current law. However, there have been no analyses of the impact on veterans in particular and what repeal could mean for demand for VA health care. As noted by Secretary of Veterans Affairs David Shulkin, a decrease in veterans' access to other sources of health coverage could lead to increases in veterans' demand for VA health care (Shane, 2017); demands on other sources of care, such as community health centers or charitable care, might also increase. Ensuring the availability of adequate resources to meet veterans' health care needs thus requires an understanding of the likely effects of ACA repeal on veterans.

Estimating the Impact of ACA Repeal on Veterans Is Complicated by Concurrent Changes in the Composition of the Veteran Population and Shifts in VA Health Care Policy

Assessment of the impact of U.S. health care reform policies on veterans must also consider the ongoing changes to the veteran population and the dynamic nature of VA health policy. The overall size of the veteran population is steadily declining at the rate of 2 percent per year, as the number of living veterans from the large World War II and Vietnam-era cohorts decreases (Eibner et al., 2015). However, even as the total number of veterans has been declining, the number of veterans using VA health care has been increasing substantially (5 percent per year averaged over the past two decades) (Eibner et al., 2015). The steady increase in veterans' use of

VA health care stems from VA policy changes that have made it easier for veterans to access VA health care, changes in the composition of the VA-eligible population, and other factors.

Changes to VA health care eligibility requirements, enrollment processes, and the availability of care have a direct impact on the number of veterans seeking VA health care. VA health care eligibility criteria often change as new health care conditions are found to be associated with military service or laws or regulations are passed to expand eligibility for certain veteran populations. For example, type 2 diabetes mellitus was recently recognized as a service-connected condition for veterans who were exposed to Agent Orange (U.S. Department of Veterans Affairs, 2016a), which increased the number of Vietnam-era veterans eligible for VA health care. A 2008 law provided enhanced eligibility for combat veterans who served in Iraq or Afghanistan, allowing these veterans to access VA care at no cost for five years after their discharge from the military (U.S. Department of Veterans Affairs, 2015). And in 2010, regulations were passed to make it easier for veterans with post-traumatic stress disorder—a signature injury from the Global War on Terror—to qualify for VA health care (U.S. Department of Veterans Affairs, 2010).

At the same time, there have been numerous changes aimed at increasing the efficiency of disability determinations and encouraging veterans to apply for benefits, including establishing a combined VA and U.S. Department of Defense disability evaluation to streamline the application process. These changes led to a sharp increase in VA disability applications, which, in turn, led to a backlog of more than 600,000 applications in 2013 (VA, 2017b). The number of backlogged claims decreased to 90,000 in 2015, adding to the population eligible for health care and increasing demand (VA, 2017b).

Over the past decade, VA has expanded its health care system to meet growing demand for care, primarily by establishing outpatient clinics that expand the system's ability to provide primary care and mental health services. Across the country, VA now operates 168 VA medical centers and more than 1,000 outpatient facilities (U.S. Department of Veterans Affairs, 2016b). Even with a growing health system, VA has had difficulty ensuring that all VA-enrolled veterans have timely and equitable access to care. In 2014, Congress passed legislation aimed at increasing veterans' access to VA health care. This law, the Veterans Access, Choice, and Accountability Act, guarantees that VA-enrolled veterans can access VA-purchased community care when their access to VA-provided care falls below certain standards (e.g., wait times longer than 30 days for an appointment or significant travel distance to a VA facility). This new program, known as the Choice program, went into effect at the end of 2014, just as many ACA provisions were starting to take effect. While initial take-up of the Choice program was slow, as the program has matured, the number of veterans receiving VA-purchased community care has increased significantly. Congress continues to consider legislative proposals to expand the program, which could have significant implications for demand for VA care.

Finally, veterans who served after September 11, 2001, currently make up a third of the nonelderly veteran population. Post-9/11 veterans differ from other service eras in enrollment and use of VA health care. A higher proportion of post-9/11 veterans use VA care than do veterans from other service eras, in part due to their enhanced eligibility for care, but also due to differences in health care needs. Because of the nature of their military service, this cohort of

6

veterans uses more care overall and more of certain types of care, including mental health care. As the post-9/11 veteran population grows as a proportion of the VA-enrolled population, demand is likely to continue to increase.

While our analysis of the impact of the ACA and efforts to repeal its provisions is unable to account for the simultaneous changes in VA health care policy, the changing VA policy context should be considered when interpreting our results.

Organization of This Report

In the next chapter, we briefly describe our methods and data sources. Complete methods and detailed analytic tables are available in Appendix A. In Chapter 3, we describe our findings on how the ACA affected nonelderly veterans' insurance status, source of coverage, and use of VA health care. Then we present our predictions for how ACA repeal and the AHCA would affect these outcomes. We present national-level estimates in the body of this report; state-level estimates are available in Appendix B. We conclude with a discussion of the implications of these findings for policymakers and VA.

2. Methods

This chapter provides a brief overview of the analytic methods used in this report. For our analyses, we used data from three surveys of the U.S. adult population: the ACS, the National Health Interview Survey (NHIS), and the Medical Expenditure Panel Survey (MEPS). A description of these surveys and thorough documentation of our methods are available in Appendix A. Where possible, our analyses draw on methods and variable definitions used in Eibner et al. (2015).

Data Sources

To analyze how the ACA has affected veterans' insurance status, we used data from two nationally representative federal household surveys: the 2013–2015 ACS and the 2011–2015 NHIS. Both surveys identify veterans by asking respondents if they have ever served on active duty in the U.S. Armed Forces, Reserves, or National Guard; neither survey collects information on whether veterans were discharged honorably.

To describe patterns of VA and total health care use by nonelderly veterans, we used the 2008–2014 MEPS. The MEPS captures detailed information about health care utilization by payer, making it a uniquely valuable data source for studying VA use in the context of veterans' use of care from non-VA sources. Although the MEPS, like the NHIS and the ACS, collects a nationally representative sample of the noninstitutionalized civilian population, it is important to note that the MEPS captures a different population of veterans from the ACS or the NHIS: The ACS and the NHIS ask whether respondents *have ever served* on active duty, whereas the MEPS asks whether respondents *have ever been honorably discharged* from active duty. Our estimates of health care use, therefore, do not reflect veterans with discharges that are other than honorable.

We restricted attention to noninstitutionalized veterans ages 19–64 at the time of the survey, and we used sampling weights provided by each survey to produce estimates that are representative of the noninstitutionalized, nonelderly veteran population. To harmonize our estimates across the different surveys used in our analysis, all estimates of totals in this report were based on 2015 population estimates from VA's VetPop2016 demographic model, which provides estimates of the veteran population by age at both the national and state levels. Because VetPop2016 estimates include veterans living in institutions (e.g., prisons or nursing homes), we scaled down all VetPop2016 estimates by 1.4 percent, which is the proportion of nonelderly veterans estimated to live in institutions in the 2015 ACS. Per-person averages estimated using survey data are multiplied by VetPop2016 estimates of the noninstitutionalized, nonelderly veteran population to produce nationwide and state-level totals.

Data Sources and Definitions

Definitions

We used data from three national surveys to estimate how current national health care reform efforts would affect veterans. None of these surveys is specifically designed to measure veterans' health care coverage and use, and different concepts may be captured by different surveys. In this report, we use the terms *VA enrollees*, *VA patients*, and *VA coverage* to be precise about these differences. These terms are defined as follows:

- o *VA enrollees:* Veterans enrolled in the Veterans Health Administration.
- o *VA patients*: Veterans who receive care at least once from VA in a year. The number of VA enrollees substantially exceeds the number of VA patients.
- o *VA coverage*: Veterans who reported having "health insurance" or "health coverage" from VA.

Data Sources

- o The **American Community Survey (ACS)** is a continuously fielded survey of the U.S. Census Bureau on a sample of the noninstitutionalized U.S. adult population, designed to collect information about education, employment, income, health insurance, disability, housing, and other characteristics, including veteran status, eras of service, and service-connected disability. Annually, the ACS samples 3.5 million residential addresses and gathers information about all members of the household.
- o The **National Health Interview Survey (NHIS)** is a nationally representative cross-sectional household interview survey of the Centers for Disease Control and Prevention, designed to collect information about individuals' health status, health behaviors, access to health care, and health insurance. Annually, the NHIS samples 35,000 households, collecting information about all members, including veteran status and era of service.
- o The survey instruments used by the ACS and NHIS are designed primarily to measure traditional health insurance coverage rather than either VA enrollee or VA patient status. When analyzing these data sources, we refer to *VA coverage* rather than *VA patients* or *VA enrollees*.
- o The **Medical Expenditure Panel Survey (MEPS)** is a panel survey of the Agency for Healthcare Research and Quality on a sample of NHIS respondents. The MEPS collects information from families and individuals about health conditions, health care use and payment, health insurance, and other topics, including whether respondents have ever been honorably discharged from the military. The MEPS does not treat VA care as a form of health insurance and does not attempt to measure VA enrollment. Instead, the MEPS allows measurement of *VA patient* status by capturing respondents' health care utilization during the two-year panel. We define *VA patients* as veterans with any care or prescriptions provided in a VA facility or paid for by VA in a calendar year.

American Community Survey

We used the ACS as our primary data source for estimating changes in health insurance coverage after implementation of the ACA's major coverage expansions.[2] The ACS has a number of advantages for studying the effect of health care reform on veterans' insurance coverage. The ACS has a very large sample size, enabling us to examine insurance status for subgroups of veterans who may be of particular interest. The ACS also contains state and substate geographic identifiers. We used geographic information in the ACS to produce state-specific estimates of insurance coverage changes following the ACA, to estimate the effects of

---

[2] We used the IPUMS ACS, which is a cleaned and harmonized version of the ACS (Ruggles et al., 2015). Some additional variables from the Census Bureau ACS files were merged into the IPUMS ACS. See Appendix A for details.

the ACA Medicaid expansion by comparing expansion and nonexpansion states, and to compare the effects of Medicaid expansion for veterans who live closer to or farther from VA facilities. In addition, the ACS collects information about service-connected disability ratings and era of service; we used these data elements along with other information in the ACS to assign respondents to potential VA priority groups.

Health coverage status and source of coverage in the ACS are measured based on respondent self-reports. Respondents are given seven response categories and an open-ended "other" response category and are instructed to select all types of health insurance or health coverage that they have at the time of the survey. We followed Census Bureau practice and categorized individuals as uninsured if they failed to report any type of insurance other than the Indian Health Service (IHS).[3] We analyzed insurance from different sources separately, allowing individuals to have multiple sources of coverage (as opposed to imposing a hierarchy to assign a primary coverage source).

Because VA is primarily an integrated health delivery system rather than an insurance program, there are some difficulties involved in measuring veterans' enrollment in and use of VA health care using surveys—such as those used in this analysis—that are designed primarily to measure health insurance coverage. Throughout this report, we distinguish between three different concepts when describing veterans' involvement with VA. *VA enrollees* refers to veterans who are enrolled in VA. While VA enrollment enables veterans to access VA care, veterans rarely disenroll from VA, and so the population of VA-enrolled veterans includes many veterans who may not have used VA care for a long time. We therefore distinguish VA enrollees from *VA patients*, who are veterans who use VA care at least once in a given calendar year.

The ACS does not directly measure either VA enrollment or VA patient status; instead, it captures whether individuals report having "health insurance or health coverage" from VA. As we discuss in Appendix A, we think that the most plausible interpretation of VA coverage as reported in the ACS is that respondents who report VA coverage are likely to have used VA care recently and thus are likely to correspond to the VA patient population; individuals who do not use VA care and have non-VA insurance are unlikely to report being covered by VA in response to survey questions about current health coverage, particularly if they have other insurance coverage and use care only from non-VA sources. This interpretation is supported by the fact that the number of VA-covered veterans in the ACS benchmarks closely to VA administrative data on the total number of VA patients. However, because we do not know of cognitive testing or audit studies that confirm this, we use the phrase *VA coverage* when referring to the population reporting health insurance or coverage from VA on the ACS. We discuss these issues at greater length in Appendix A.

---

[3] The IHS provides care to qualifying individuals, but Census Bureau health insurance statistics do not count IHS coverage as health insurance because many IHS enrollees do not have access to comprehensive health care (Barnett and Vornovitsky, 2016).

National Health Interview Survey

We used the NHIS to remedy certain limitations of the ACS for measuring insurance status. The ACS relies on respondent self-reports to correctly identify the source of insurance, and respondents are known to underreport Medicaid coverage and overreport direct-purchase coverage (Lynch and Kenney, 2011). The NHIS is a more-accurate data source for identifying Americans' sources of health insurance coverage, thanks to extensive follow-up questions and logical edits built into the survey. Also unlike the ACS, the NHIS distinguishes between Marketplace and non-Marketplace direct-purchase coverage, and so we relied on the NHIS to measure take-up of Marketplace coverage by veterans. The NHIS also collects detailed information about respondents' health conditions, and we used this information to estimate the proportion of nonelderly veterans with preexisting conditions that would make it difficult to purchase nongroup coverage if repeal of the ACA allowed insurers to return to pre-ACA practices of medical underwriting.

Our use of the NHIS in this study was limited, however, because the NHIS has a much smaller sample size than the ACS. The NHIS also does not collect information about service-connected disability, making it infeasible to assign veterans in the NHIS to priority groups. Finally, state codes and substate geographic information are not available in the public-use NHIS, making it unsuitable for analyzing the effects of Medicaid expansion or other geographic differences. Instead, the primary function of the NHIS in this study is to examine whether the changes in coverage by source that we estimate using the ACS were driven by reporting errors. We did not find any estimates of post-ACA coverage changes in the NHIS that differ meaningfully from our estimates in the ACS; NHIS coverage estimates are reported in Appendix A.

Medical Expenditure Panel Survey

We used data from the 2008–2014 MEPS to describe patterns of VA use among the nonelderly veteran population. We estimated the relationship between veterans' health care use from VA and other sources and their individual characteristics, including age, income, health status, and non-VA insurance coverage; these estimates were an important input into our analysis of ACA repeal. In five interviews covering two years of health care use, the MEPS collects self-reported event histories of health care use in addition to a range of demographic, insurance coverage, and economic variables. In particular, respondents are asked to identify where they received care, who they received care from, and how the care was paid for. The MEPS then uses follow-back interviews with a sample of health care providers to corroborate these self-reports. Information from the household and provider interviews is synthesized into a series of event files that provide each respondent's history of health care use over the two-year panel.

Unlike the ACS and the NHIS, the MEPS does not treat VA as a form of health insurance. The concept of *VA coverage* that we observe in the ACS is thus not observable in the MEPS. Instead, the MEPS provides us with observations of *VA patient* status and *VA use*. We defined *VA use* as the number of health care events provided by a VA provider or paid for by VA. VA patients are veterans who use VA care once or more in a calendar year. We constructed measures of annual VA use for each respondent by counting the number of health care events in three categories of care: office-based visits, inpatient surgery, and prescription drugs obtained. All our estimates of the quantity of health care used by veterans thus refer to counts of health care events (numbers of office visits, surgeries, or prescriptions filled) per year. Our approach to measuring VA use followed as closely as possible the methods developed in Eibner et al. (2015). Additional details and summary statistics are presented in Appendix A.

Statistical Methods

We used several different types of statistical models to analyze our three data sources for this study. This section provides a brief overview; key points are highlighted in Table 2.1. Additional information is presented as we discuss our results, and detailed descriptions of our methods are presented in Appendix A.

Table 2.1. Overview of Data Sources, Populations, and Methods Used in This Study

Analysis	Data Source	Population of Interest	Method
Changes in insurance coverage between 2013 and 2015	2013–2015 ACS	Noninstitutionalized, nonelderly veterans	Before-after (logistic regression)
Effects of Medicaid expansion	2013–2015 ACS	Noninstitutionalized, nonelderly veterans with family income below 138 percent of FPL	Differences in differences (logistic regression)
VA and total health care use and reliance, by demographics and insurance status	2008–2014 MEPS	Noninstitutionalized, nonelderly veterans; noninstitutionalized, nonelderly VA patients	Cross-sectional Poisson regression
Predicted coverage changes under ACA repeal or the AHCA	2013–2015 ACS; RAND COMPARE; 2015 NHIS	Noninstitutionalized, nonelderly veterans	Calculate predicted percentage change in uninsurance rate by age, income, and health status; multiply by baseline scenario uninsurance rate
Effects of ACA repeal or the AHCA on VA and total health care use	2008–2014 MEPS	Noninstitutionalized, nonelderly veterans	Use predicted coverage changes and Poisson regression estimates to calculate average health care use of veterans losing insurance; apply semi-elasticities derived from Shen et al. (2008) to predict change in VA and total health care use
Prevalence of declinable preexisting conditions	2015 NHIS	Noninstitutionalized, nonelderly veterans	Apply definition of preexisting conditions used in Claxton et al. (2016); logistic regression

NOTE: COMPARE = Comprehensive Assessment of Reform Efforts.

12

To estimate how veterans' health insurance coverage has changed since ACA implementation, we used logistic regression to control for veterans' ages, genders, races/ethnicities, and service eras. It is necessary to control for these confounding factors because many Vietnam-era veterans turned 65 between 2013 and 2015; compared with the 2013 nonelderly veteran population, the 2015 nonelderly veteran population is younger, more likely to be female, more likely to be nonwhite or Hispanic, and more likely to have completed military service in the post-9/11 era. ACS data on veterans from before 2013 are not comparable to current data, so our analysis of the ACS uses pooled data from 2013–2015 and focuses largely on changes between 2013 and 2015 (Holder and Raglin, 2014). To estimate changes in coverage in the NHIS, we pooled data from 2011–2015 and used 2011–2013 as a baseline period to obtain a larger sample size; changes estimated using only 2013–2015 data were similar but less precise. In models estimating adjusted changes in coverage over time, we used the survey design variables provided by each survey to conduct statistical inference. We also used this estimation framework to examine changes in coverage for several subpopulations of interest: veterans gaining Medicaid eligibility due to the ACA, previously Medicaid-eligible veterans, and veterans with different VA priority groups.

Besides estimating changes in coverage that occurred after ACA implementation, we were able to use a differences-in-differences approach to estimate the effects of Medicaid expansion on nonelderly veterans' insurance coverage. Specifically, we used Medicaid nonexpansion states as a control group for Medicaid expansion states and compared the adjusted changes in coverage for low-income adults targeted by the Medicaid expansion (family income below 138 percent of FPL) from 2013 to 2015 between the two groups of states. The difference in the changes observed in each group of states can be attributed to Medicaid expansion under the assumption that outcomes would have evolved similarly in the absence of Medicaid expansion. In differences-in-differences estimates and other regression models in which the key variables of interest vary at the state level, we used standard errors clustered on state to conduct statistical inference. As with our before-after estimates of changes in coverage between 2013 and 2015, we estimated differences-in-differences models for both the overall population of nonelderly low-income veterans and for subgroups of veterans. In particular, we used a differences-in-differences model to estimate the effect of Medicaid expansion separately for veterans who live near VA facilities and for veterans who live farther from VA facilities.

To characterize how veterans' use of VA health care and their total use of health care from all payers (including VA) varied with individual characteristics, we estimated Poisson regression models for annual VA use and total use of health care. To describe patterns of VA use and reliance for VA patients, we restricted the estimation sample to VA patients. Covariates used in these models included age, gender, race/ethnicity, income, health status, and whether individuals were uninsured for the full calendar year (as opposed to being covered by non-VA health insurance at some time during the year). Adjusted levels of VA and total health care use for insured and uninsured veterans were calculated as predicted outcomes from these Poisson regression models. Adjusted VA reliance was defined as the ratio of predicted VA use to predicted total use.

To analyze the impact of ACA repeal or reforms similar to the AHCA on nonelderly veterans' use of VA health care, we specified a model linking changes in non-VA insurance coverage to changes in VA and total health care use. As inputs to this analysis, we used before-after ACS estimates and model output from the RAND COMPARE model's analysis of the AHCA to define the predicted percentage change in the uninsured population within eight subgroups of veterans, defined by age, income, and health status. We applied these predicted percentage changes to a baseline scenario representing health insurance coverage rates and health care use in each subgroup for the 2015 nonelderly veteran population: Baseline health insurance coverage was estimated using the ACS and NHIS, while baseline health care use was predicted using our Poisson regression estimates from the 2008–2014 MEPS. These calculations yielded an estimate of the average VA and total health care use for veterans anticipated to lose (or gain) insurance coverage under each scenario. We then used estimates from the peer-reviewed research literature to predict the changes in VA and total health care utilization that would result from these changes in insurance coverage.

We note that our analysis of the AHCA is driven by anticipated changes in the number of uninsured veterans, using model results that are driven largely by removal of coverage mandates, changes to the Marketplaces, and reductions in Medicaid eligibility and funding. Our quantitative estimates of current ACA repeal proposals thus do not capture the effects of other potentially important changes proposed as part of ACA repeal, including changes to the essential health benefits and other possible consequences of expanded state waiver authority; in Chapter 4, we provide a qualitative discussion of selected other provisions and their possible impacts on veterans. Because the AHCA and related legislation have included changes that might make it more difficult for some individuals with preexisting health conditions to purchase comprehensive health insurance, we used an algorithm developed by the Kaiser Family Foundation to calculate the proportion of nonelderly veterans with preexisting conditions that would have prevented them from purchasing nongroup insurance in the pre-ACA market (Claxton et al., 2016).

Finally, we produced state-specific estimates of adjusted changes in coverage for 30 states with large populations of nonelderly veterans. Adjusted coverage estimates are estimated using interacted versions of our main before-after logistic regression model, in which the change in coverage between 2013 and 2015 varies freely across states. We also used VetPop2016 estimates of the age structure of each state's veteran population, along with COMPARE estimates of the effects of the AHCA by age and state Medicaid expansion status, to calculate state-specific changes in VA use that would result from coverage changes similar to those anticipated under the AHCA in 2020 and 2026. These state-specific estimates are available as an online appendix and are described in greater detail in Appendix B (see www.rand.org/t/RR1955 for downloads).

3. After the ACA, Fewer Nonelderly Veterans Were Uninsured, and More Reported Medicaid, Private, and VA Coverage

Nonelderly Veterans Had Higher Rates of Insurance Coverage After the ACA Than Before

More nonelderly veterans had insurance coverage after the ACA than before; using data from the U.S. Census Bureau, we found that the proportion of uninsured nonelderly veterans fell from 9.1 percent in 2013 to 5.8 percent in 2015, after adjusting for changes in the distribution of age, gender, race/ethnicity, and service era. Our findings confirm those previously reported by the Urban Institute (Haley, Kenney, and Gates, 2017), which also found that reductions in veteran uninsurance were accompanied by reductions in self-reports of unmet health care needs.

Increases in insurance coverage from both public and private sources contributed to the reduction in uninsurance among nonelderly veterans (Figure 3.1). The adjusted 2.6-percentage-point increase in Medicaid coverage was similar to the overall increase in private coverage, which included increases in both employer-sponsored insurance (ESI) and direct-purchase coverage. While not shown, nonelderly veterans had slightly lower rates of insurance coverage from TRICARE in 2015 than in 2013 after adjusting for age and service era (detailed tables available in Appendix A).

Figure 3.1. Uninsurance and Coverage by Source for Nonelderly Veterans, Adjusted for Age and Service Era

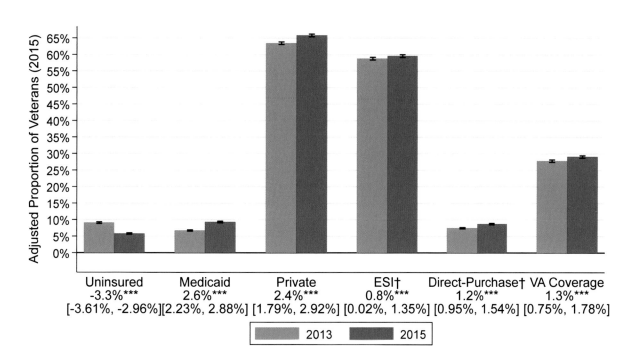

SOURCES: Authors' calculations, 2013 and 2015 IPUMS ACS.

NOTES: ESI = employer-sponsored insurance.
† Direct-purchase coverage includes both Marketplace coverage and other non-Marketplace nongroup coverage. Respondents are counted as having private coverage if they report either ESI or direct-purchase coverage. Respondents may report more than one coverage type, and so changes in ESI and direct-purchase may not sum to the change in private coverage.
Adjusted differences between 2015 and 2013 coverage rate are reported below bar labels. The 95-percent confidence interval for difference is reported in brackets. * $p < 0.10$, ** $p < 0.05$, *** $p < 0.01$. Error bars depict 95-percent confidence intervals for adjusted coverage rate. Adjusted coverage rates and differences represent predictions from logistic regressions controlling for age, race/ethnicity, gender, and service era averaged over the 2015 distribution of sample characteristics. See Appendix A for coefficient estimates and further details.

Both the Marketplaces and the Medicaid Expansion Contributed to Coverage Gains for Nonelderly Veterans

We analyzed the ACS and the NHIS to learn more about which ACA provisions may have led to the coverage increases observed between 2013 and 2015. Because the ACS does not distinguish between Marketplace plans and other direct-purchase coverage, we used the NHIS to measure the proportion of nonelderly veterans with Marketplace coverage. By 2015, 2.4 percent of nonelderly veterans were enrolled in Marketplace plans. As with the broader nonelderly population, enrollment in Marketplace coverage increased sharply with age. While just 1.1 percent of post-9/11 veterans had Marketplace coverage in 2015, 4.7 percent of Vietnam-era veterans had Marketplace coverage in 2015. The proportion of nonelderly veterans estimated to have Marketplace coverage in the NHIS as of 2015 was slightly larger than the overall increase in direct-purchase coverage observed between 2013 and 2015, suggesting that some nonelderly veterans with Marketplace coverage might have purchased nongroup coverage in the absence of the ACA; while the NHIS shows a larger adjusted increase in direct-purchase coverage (2.0 percentage points) than we estimated in the ACS (1.2 percentage points), the NHIS estimate is much less precise due to the smaller sample size in that survey and does not differ from the ACS estimate by a statistically significant margin.

We used the ACS to estimate the effect of the Medicaid expansion by comparing changes in coverage from 2013 to 2015 between expansion and nonexpansion states (see Table 3.1). The proportion of nonelderly veterans with no health insurance declined more sharply in Medicaid expansion states than in nonexpansion states—by 1.4 percentage points after adjusting for age, gender, race/ethnicity, and service era. These results are consistent with estimates previously reported by the Urban Institute (Haley, Kenney, and Gates, 2017). Among nonelderly veterans in the income range targeted by the Medicaid expansion (family income below 138 percent of FPL), the uninsurance rate fell by an adjusted 4.4 percentage points more in Medicaid expansion states than in nonexpansion states between 2013 and 2015.

Low-income veterans in expansion states had an adjusted 8.4-percentage-point increase in the probability of having Medicaid coverage relative to nonexpansion states, but they also had an adjusted 2.5-percentage-point decrease in the probability of having private coverage. We did not find any differences due to Medicaid expansion in the likelihood of having employer-sponsored insurance, but we did find that low-income veterans in expansion states were less likely to have direct-purchase coverage (including Marketplace coverage). This is likely explained by the fact that in nonexpansion states, low-income adults with family income above 100 percent of FPL are eligible for Marketplace subsidies.

Table 3.1. Effects of Medicaid Expansion on Uninsurance and Source of Coverage for Nonelderly Veterans (2015)

	Uninsured	Medicaid	Private	ESI	Direct Purchase
Medicaid expansion effect for all nonelderly veterans	−1.4%***	2.4%***	−0.7%	−0.4%	−0.4
	[−1.9%, −0.9%]	[1.6%, 3.2%]	[−1.7%, 0.3%]	[−1.4%, 0.6%]	[−1.0%, 0.3%]
Medicaid expansion effect for nonelderly veterans with family income below 138 percent of FPL	−4.4%***	8.4%***	−2.5%**	−0.9%	−1.9%**
	[−6.3%, −2.4%]	[5.1%, 11.6%]	[−4.6%, −0.4%]	[−3.0%, 1.1%]	[−3.4%, −0.4%]

SOURCE: Authors' calculations, 2013–2015 IPUMS ACS.
NOTES: * $p < 0.10$, ** $p < 0.05$, *** $p < 0.01$. This table reports marginal effects of state Medicaid expansion interacted with an indicator for the year 2015 from separate logistic regressions of coverage on state and year fixed effects, age, gender, race/ethnicity, and service-era controls, as well as interactions between state Medicaid expansion and indicators for the years 2014 and 2015. Marginal effects are calculated for the 2015 distribution of sample characteristics. See Appendix A for details.

Medicaid expansion increased insurance coverage through two distinct channels: by expanding Medicaid eligibility to all adults with family income below 138 percent of FPL, regardless of family structure, and by encouraging Medicaid take-up among previously eligible but uninsured adults. To encourage take-up, the ACA contained many measures intended to facilitate Medicaid enrollment, and additional factors, such as the publicity surrounding ACA implementation and the individual mandate, may also have served to increase Medicaid enrollment among previously eligible adults in both expansion and nonexpansion states. For the general adult population, roughly half of the gains in coverage due to Medicaid occurred among previously eligible adults, with the other half attributable to expanded eligibility (Frean, Gruber, and Sommers, 2017). A rollback of Medicaid expansion would, by definition, reduce Medicaid coverage for newly eligible veterans but may not have direct impacts on the previously eligible, newly enrolled population. In contrast, changes to Medicaid enrollment procedures or eligibility standards that make enrollment more onerous (for example, the requirement in the House and Senate bills that states verify income eligibility for Medicaid at least every six months) might decrease enrollment among both newly and previously eligible adults.

To gain further insight into the mechanisms through which the ACA Medicaid expansion may have reduced uninsurance among nonelderly veterans, we used ACS data on family income to impute Medicaid eligibility for nonelderly veterans, distinguishing between those who would have been eligible for Medicaid under each state's income limits in 2013 (*previously eligible* veterans) and those who gained Medicaid eligibility as a result of Medicaid expansion under the ACA (*newly eligible* veterans).[4] We then estimated changes in insurance coverage between 2013 and 2015 for the previously eligible and newly eligible veteran populations, adjusting for age, gender, race/ethnicity, and service era.

In the 29 states (including the District of Columbia) that had implemented the ACA's Medicaid expansion by June 2015, we estimated that 19.5 percent of nonelderly veterans were eligible for Medicaid in 2015, compared with 10.1 percent who were eligible for Medicaid in 2013, before the ACA. In these states, nonelderly veterans who were eligible for Medicaid in 2015 were split almost evenly between previously eligible (10 percent of nonelderly veterans) and those who were newly eligible (9.2 percent of nonelderly veterans). In the remaining 22 states, we estimated that just 4 percent of nonelderly veterans were eligible for Medicaid in 2015 under the income limits in effect on July 1, 2015, a small increase from the 3.5 percent who were eligible in 2013. As discussed by Haley, Kenney, and Gates (2017), the low levels of Medicaid eligibility in nonexpansion states mean that a sizable number of uninsured nonelderly veterans would stand to gain coverage if those states expanded Medicaid: The researchers estimated that one in five uninsured nonelderly veterans would gain Medicaid eligibility if all nonexpansion states implemented the expansion.

Medicaid-eligible veterans in both expansion and nonexpansion states experienced meaningful reductions in uninsurance between 2013 and 2015, but the magnitude of the reductions varied with state expansion status and pre-ACA eligibility. In Medicaid expansion states, both previously eligible and newly eligible nonelderly veterans experienced large reductions in uninsurance between 2013 and 2015. The adjusted probability of being uninsured

---

[4] See Appendix A for details.

fell by 12 percentage points for newly eligible nonelderly veterans and by 7.7 percentage points for previously eligible veterans. The decline in uninsurance was statistically significantly larger for newly eligible veterans, a pattern similar to that documented by Frean, Gruber, and Sommers (2017) for the overall population under age 65.[5] We also found a smaller, but significant, decline in uninsurance (–3.4 percentage points) and an increase in Medicaid coverage (4.7 percentage points) for the previously eligible population in nonexpansion states.

Medicaid Expansion Led to Increased Insurance Coverage for Veterans Who Live Far from VA Care

VA-eligible veterans who live far from VA facilities may be less likely to enroll in and use VA care than those who live closer to a VA facility. Indeed, VA has recently focused on expanding access through the Choice program to veterans living farther than 40 miles from a VA facility (Veterans Access, Choice, and Accountability Act of 2014). We assessed whether veterans living far from a VA facility were more or less likely to gain insurance coverage after the ACA than were veterans living close to a VA facility. Although the ACS does not provide detailed location information on respondents to preserve confidentiality, the public-use ACS does assign respondents to more than 2,000 substate geographic areas known as Public Use Microdata Areas (PUMAs). For each PUMA in the United States, we calculated the distance from the PUMA centroid to the nearest VA Medical Center (VAMC) and the nearest VA outpatient facility; we assigned this distance to each veteran in the PUMA as a rough proxy for distance to VA facilities. Weighted by the nonelderly veteran population, the median distance from a PUMA centroid to a VAMC was 25 miles, and the median distance from a PUMA centroid to an outpatient facility was 12 miles. We categorized veterans as living far from a VA facility if they lived farther than the median distance that veterans live from a VAMC *and* farther than the median distance from an outpatient facility.[6] In 2015, one in three nonelderly veterans was living in an area that was far from a VA facility under this definition. Although it might have been ideal to use the 40-mile threshold established by the Choice Act, we found that only 5 percent of nonelderly veterans lived in an area that was 40 miles or more from any VA facilities, and so estimates for this group were too imprecise to be informative.

On a nationwide basis, we did not find evidence that changes in insurance coverage between 2013 and 2015 varied with distance from VA facilities. We did, however, find that the ACA Medicaid expansion had larger effects on the insurance status of veterans who live far from VA facilities. Figure 3.2 shows the estimated effects of the Medicaid expansion on veterans' insurance coverage for low-income veterans in the income range targeted by the Medicaid expansion (below 138 percent of FPL) who live closer to versus farther from a VA facility.

---

[5] See Appendix A for estimates.

[6] There is no universally accepted standard for geographic access to health care providers. However, many states have established quantitative limits to regulate provider network adequacy (Health Affairs, 2016). While different states take different approaches, the bifurcated approach we take here (setting one threshold for hospitals and a lower threshold for primary care) is currently used as part of California's provider network adequacy standard. California uses a distance threshold of 15 miles for primary care and mental health providers and a threshold of 30 miles for specialists and hospitals (California Department of Insurance, undated).

Medicaid expansion reduced the probability of uninsurance for both groups of veterans. Although the effect of Medicaid expansion on uninsurance appears to be larger for veterans living farther from VA facilities, we did not find that the effect of Medicaid expansion on the probability of being uninsured differed between the two groups by a statistically significant margin.

However, when we consider insurance from non-VA sources, we found that Medicaid expansion differentially reduced the probability that low-income veterans in the income range targeted by the Medicaid expansion (below 138 percent of FPL) living far from VA facilities lacked non-VA insurance. Medicaid expansion reduced non-VA uninsurance by an adjusted 5.7 percentage points for low-income veterans living close to VA facilities and by an adjusted 11.3 percentage points for low-income veterans living far from VA facilities.[7] This differential increase in non-VA insurance coverage was accounted for by greater take-up of Medicaid coverage by veterans living far from VA facilities.

---

[7] See Appendix A for estimates.

Figure 3.2. Effects of Medicaid Expansion on Insurance Status and VA Coverage, Nonelderly Veterans with Family Income Below 138 Percent of FPL, by Distance to Nearest VA Facilities

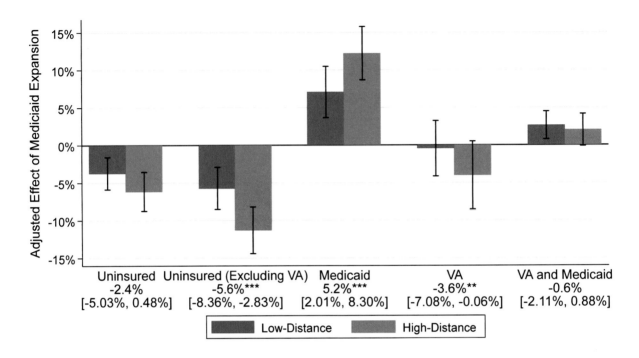

SOURCE: Authors' calculations, 2013–2015 IPUMS ACS.

NOTES: This figure depicts marginal effects, with 95-percent confidence intervals, of Medicaid expansion on insurance coverage. The differences (95-percent confidence interval) between low-distance and high-distance marginal effects are reported below the bar labels. * $p < 0.10$, ** $p < 0.05$, *** $p < 0.01$. The significance of difference was assessed based on regression coefficients. Medicaid expansion effects were estimated using logistic regressions controlling for age, race/ethnicity, gender, service era, and fixed effects for state and year. State and year fixed effects were interacted with distance from VA. See Appendix A for coefficient estimates and further details. This model allows the effect of Medicaid expansion to vary with veterans' distance from VA facilities. The distance from VA facilities was measured from the centroid of the PUMA. Veterans are classified as high distance if they live in a PUMA that is more than 12 miles from a VA outpatient facility and more than 25 miles from a VAMC; they are classified as low distance otherwise. These thresholds are the median population-weighted distances to each type of VA facility for nonelderly veterans.

State-Specific Estimates Show That Increases in the Number of Insured Veterans Were Widespread, with the Largest Increases Concentrated in Medicaid Expansion States

In Appendix B, we present state-level estimates of the number of veterans uninsured or covered by each of the insurance sources examined previously, as well as estimates of the change in insurance status between 2013 and 2015, adjusted for age, gender, race/ethnicity, and service era. We found that the largest reductions in the proportion of veterans without insurance were concentrated in Medicaid expansion states, particularly Oregon, Arkansas, Nevada, Kentucky, and Washington. We present estimates for 30 states in Appendix B, including 19 expansion states and 11 nonexpansion states.

More VA-Enrolled Veterans Had Non-VA Insurance Coverage Following ACA Implementation, Particularly Medicaid

With the ACA's coverage expansions, some uninsured nonelderly veterans who were eligible for VA health care may have chosen to enroll in VA health care to obtain qualifying coverage and avoid individual-mandate penalties. Other uninsured low-income veterans, including some who were previously enrolled in VA health care or expected to use VA health care in the future, may have qualified for tax credits to purchase coverage in insurance Marketplaces, or they may have lived in states that opted to expand Medicaid. These individuals may have transitioned away from the VA health care system to other providers to receive some or all of their care (Frakt, Hanchate, and Pizer, 2015). These new options for health coverage may have been especially valuable for VA-enrolled veterans who lived far from a VA facility or otherwise had difficulty accessing VA care, as VA initiatives to expand access to care, such as the Choice program, had not yet been implemented. However, as mentioned previously, there were other concurrent VA policy changes during this period that may have affected VA coverage for nonelderly veterans.

We used data from the 2013–2015 ACS to describe changes in the proportion of nonelderly veterans reporting VA coverage, as well as changes in patterns of dual VA/non-VA coverage and the proportion of veterans reporting only VA coverage. Because we did not have access to VA data on enrollees or patients, our estimates may be an undercount of the number of nonelderly veterans affected by these changes. Undercounting in the ACS results from misreporting by respondents and limitations in reaching individuals not living in housing units or group quarters.

Nonelderly Veterans Gained VA Coverage Between 2013 and 2015

More nonelderly veterans reported having VA health coverage in 2015 (an adjusted 29.1 percent) compared with 2013 (an adjusted 27.8 percent). Because most veterans who are enrolled in VA health care also have another source of health coverage, such as Medicare or private insurance, we were also interested in changes in dual VA and non-VA coverage. Among nonelderly veterans who reported having VA coverage, the share that reported VA coverage as their only source of health coverage decreased by 1.3 percentage points after the ACA, while the share that reported having both VA coverage and Medicaid increased by 2.7 percentage points (Figure 3.3). There was not a significant difference in the proportion of veterans reporting having both VA coverage and private health insurance.

Figure 3.3. Change in VA Coverage and Non-VA Insurance for VA-Covered Nonelderly Veterans, Adjusted by Age and Service Era

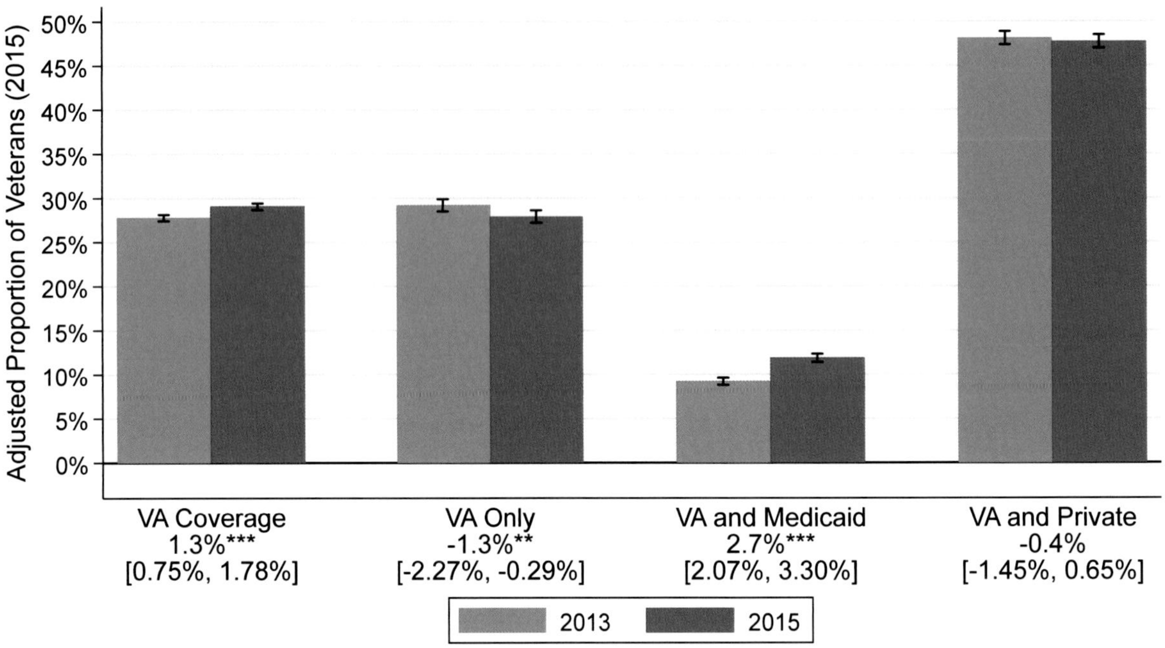

SOURCE: Authors' calculations, 2013–2015 IPUMS ACS.

NOTES: Proportions with VA coverage were calculated among all nonelderly veterans. Proportions with VA only, VA and Medicaid, and VA and private coverage were calculated among nonelderly veterans reporting VA coverage. *VA only* coverage includes individuals reporting VA coverage with no other health insurance. *VA and Medicaid* coverage includes individuals reporting both VA and Medicaid coverage. *VA and private* coverage includes individuals reporting both VA and private coverage. Adjusted differences between 2015 and 2013 coverage rates are reported below bar labels. The 95-percent confidence interval for difference is reported in brackets. * $p < 0.10$, ** $p < 0.05$, *** $p < 0.01$. Error bars depict 95-percent confidence intervals for the adjusted coverage rate. Adjusted coverage rates and differences represent predictions from logistic regressions controlling for age, race/ethnicity, gender, and service era. See Appendix A for coefficient estimates and further details.

VA Coverage Changes Differed After the ACA for Different Groups of Veterans

Changes in VA coverage after the ACA differed significantly by VA enrollment priority group (Table 3.2). Low-priority–group veterans (with higher incomes) had the largest absolute reduction in uninsurance (9.0-percent decrease), primarily driven by increases in VA coverage and private insurance coverage. High-priority–group low-income veterans also had a significant reduction in uninsurance (7.0-percent decrease). However, changes in VA coverage for this group were smaller than for higher-income veterans, and reductions in uninsurance were instead driven primarily by increases in Medicaid coverage. High-priority–group veterans with service-connected disabilities experienced more-muted reductions in uninsurance than did low-income and low-priority–group veterans, reflecting, in part, the fact that veterans with service-connected disabilities were already less likely to be uninsured prior to ACA implementation.

Table 3.2. Change in Uninsurance and VA Coverage Among Nonelderly VA-Eligible Veterans Between 2013 and 2015, by Estimated VA Enrollment Priority Group

	Uninsured	VA Coverage	VA Only	VA and Medicaid	VA and Private
High-priority–group veterans with service-connected disabilities (priority groups 1–4, 6)	−0.8%*** [−1.1%, −0.5%]	−0.03% [−1.1%, 1.0%]	−0.5% [−1.2%, 0.3%]	1.5%*** [1.0%, 1.9%]	−1.4%*** [−2.3%, −0.5%]
High-priority–group, low-income veterans (priority group 5)	−7.0%*** [−8.1%, −6.0%]	1.6%** [0.4%, 2.9%]	−0.9%** [−1.7%, −0.1%]	3.1%*** [2.4%, 3.8%]	0.5% [−0.2%, 1.3%]
Low-priority–group veterans (priority groups 7–8d)	−9.0%*** [−10.2%, −7.7%]	14.6%*** [12.8%, 16.4%]	3.5%*** [2.0%, 5.0%]	−0.03% [−0.4%, 0.4%]	11.0%*** [9.5%, 12.5%]

SOURCE: Authors' calculations, 2013–2015 IPUMS ACS.
NOTES: * $p < 0.10$, ** $p < 0.05$, *** $p < 0.01$. *VA only* coverage includes individuals reporting VA coverage with no other health insurance. *VA and Medicaid* coverage includes individuals reporting both VA and Medicaid coverage. *VA and private* includes individuals reporting both VA and private coverage. The population used to calculate all changes in rates includes all nonelderly veterans.
This table reports adjusted changes from 2013 to 2015 fully interacted with VA priority group categories. Each column reports estimates from a separate logistic regression of coverage on state and year fixed effects and age, gender, race/ethnicity, and service-era controls, in addition to interactions between priority group categories and indicators for the years 2014 and 2015. Marginal effects are calculated for the 2015 distribution of sample characteristics within each priority group category. See Appendix A for details.

VA coverage for high-priority–group veterans with service-connected disabilities did not change between 2013 and 2015 after adjusting for age and service era. However, we found that high-priority–group veterans became less likely to have only VA coverage, with increases in dual coverage driven by VA-Medicaid dual enrollment. We observed increased VA-Medicaid dual enrollment for both disabled veterans and low-income veterans. For low-priority–group VA-eligible veterans, a different pattern emerged. There was a moderately large increase of 3.5 percentage points in the proportion with only VA coverage and a large increase (11 percentage points) in the proportion with both VA coverage and private coverage.

We also examined whether the effect of the Medicaid expansion on VA coverage varied with veterans' distance to VA facilities. These estimates were presented in Figure 3.2. We did not find that Medicaid expansion resulted in a differentially larger increase in VA-Medicaid dual enrollment for veterans living far from VA facilities compared with veterans living closer to VA facilities. Compared with veterans living a similar distance from VA in nonexpansion states, Medicaid expansion increased the probability of VA-Medicaid dual enrollment by 2.6 percentage points for veterans near VA facilities and by 2.0 percentage points for veterans far from VA facilities. The difference between these Medicaid expansion effects was not statistically significant. However, there is some suggestive evidence that Medicaid expansion reduced the probability of VA coverage for low-income veterans living far from VA facilities, while

Medicaid expansion had no effect on VA coverage for veterans living close to VA facilities.[8] This provides some evidence that Medicaid coverage made available through the Medicaid expansion provided veterans with a substitute for VA coverage. Even though the Medicaid expansion reduced VA coverage for veterans living far from VA facilities (in comparison with similar veterans in nonexpansion states), the increase in Medicaid coverage for veterans living far from VA facilities was large enough to offset this reduction in VA coverage, meaning that the rate of uninsurance declined more sharply for veterans in expansion states even as they were also less likely to be covered through VA.

VA Coverage Increased in Most States, with Changes in Dual Enrollment Differing by State Medicaid Expansion Status

Appendix B also reports estimates of the adjusted change in VA coverage and different types of dual enrollment. Most states saw an increase in VA coverage after adjustment for age and service era, with the largest increases observed in Alabama, Louisiana, Tennessee, Florida, and Arizona. As noted previously, there has long been a trend of increased VA enrollment for reasons unrelated to the ACA, so we cannot clearly attribute this pattern to the ACA. In Louisiana[9] and five nonexpansion states, the proportion of veterans with VA coverage alone (no non-VA coverage) rose by more than 1 percentage point. Increases in VA-Medicaid dual enrollment were concentrated in Medicaid expansion states. Increases in VA-private dual enrollment, which were also apparent in most states, were not significantly correlated with Medicaid expansion status.[10]

Increases in Non-VA Insurance Coverage May Have Changed Patterns of VA Utilization

Our analysis of the ACS confirmed previously reported findings that the proportion of nonelderly veterans without health insurance fell after the ACA's major coverage expansions took effect in 2014 (Haley, Kenney, and Gates, 2017). Both Medicaid and private insurance coverage increased for nonelderly veterans between 2013 and 2015. Gains in private coverage were driven by direct-purchase coverage, which includes Marketplace coverage. Increases in Medicaid coverage were sharpest for newly eligible veterans in expansion states, but previously eligible veterans in both expansion and nonexpansion states also were more likely to be covered by Medicaid in 2015 than in 2013.

---

[8] The marginal effect of Medicaid expansion on VA coverage for high-distance veterans is not significant at the 5-percent level, but it is significant at the 10-percent level ($p = 0.081$). It is possible for the effect for high-distance veterans to be significantly different from the effect for low-distance veterans (which is less than zero) but not significantly different from zero if the two estimated marginal effects are positively correlated.

[9] Louisiana's Medicaid expansion took effect in 2016, and we have accordingly coded it as a nonexpansion state for our empirical analysis.

[10] Significance was assessed using a rank correlation between state Medicaid expansion status and the point estimate for the adjusted change in coverage.

We did not have an adequate control group to isolate the effect of the Marketplaces, premium subsidies, and other nationwide reforms to the individual market. However, the 22 states that had not expanded Medicaid before late 2015 provide a valuable control group that allowed us to estimate the effect of Medicaid expansion on veterans' insurance status and sources of insurance. Medicaid expansion reduced the rate of uninsurance for low-income veterans in the income range targeted by the expansion. Low-income veterans who live far from VA facilities experienced particularly large gains in Medicaid coverage and reductions in uninsurance as a result of Medicaid expansion.

VA coverage for nonelderly veterans also increased between 2013 and 2015. Although we found an adjusted increase in VA coverage between 2013 and 2015, VA enrollment had been rising steadily before the ACA, making it unclear how much of this increase should be attributed to the ACA. Similarly, we did not find any evidence that Medicaid expansion affected VA coverage for low-income veterans.

To understand the effects of the ACA on demand for VA care, we also examined patterns of non-VA insurance coverage among VA-covered nonelderly veterans. While VA coverage increased nationwide, we found that the overall increase in coverage between 2013 and 2015 was driven by veterans with either private insurance or Medicaid in addition to VA coverage; there was no adjusted change in the proportion of nonelderly veterans with only VA coverage. The proportion of VA-covered nonelderly veterans who lacked non-VA insurance fell, while the proportion with Medicaid coverage in addition to VA coverage rose. We found that these increases in VA-Medicaid dual enrollment were larger in Medicaid expansion states. Our analysis of coverage changes by priority group showed significant increases in VA-Medicaid dual enrollment for both low-income eligible veterans (priority group 5) and disabled veterans (priority groups 1–4 and 6).

In short, implementation of the ACA was followed by reductions in the number of veterans who lacked any form of health insurance and increases in the number of VA-covered veterans who were dually enrolled in some non-VA source of insurance. Given these increases in non-VA insurance coverage, one might expect to see changes in veterans' patterns of health care utilization, including a shift from VA to non-VA providers. However, it is not yet possible to estimate the effect of the ACA on VA health care use with publicly available data from the period after the ACA was fully implemented. The MEPS is the best publicly available data source for understanding veterans' health care use, but its relatively small single-year veteran sample size limits the types of analyses that are possible. In addition, at the time of this analysis, only data through 2014 were available. Our estimates of differences in use between 2014 and earlier years were too imprecise to be informative, and we do not report them in this study.

This meant that we were not able to directly measure the impact of the ACA on VA patients' use of VA health care. Instead, we used the 2008–2014 MEPS to model the relationship between non-VA health coverage, individual characteristics, and veterans' use of health care from VA and other sources; estimates from these statistical models are used as an input into our analysis of ACA repeal. Our estimates of these models also allowed us to characterize how veterans use both VA and non-VA care and how patterns of health care use vary with key demographic characteristics. We present descriptive evidence on veterans' health care use before turning to our analysis of changes that might result from ACA repeal; additional estimates and methods are presented in Appendix A.

Nonelderly Veterans Receive Most of Their Health Care from Non-VA Providers, Even If They Are VA Patients

We used data from the 2008–2014 MEPS to describe nonelderly veterans' use of VA and other health care. In contrast with the other surveys analyzed in this study, the MEPS directly measures health care paid for or provided by VA but does not treat VA enrollment or patient status as a form of health insurance. We defined *VA patients* as nonelderly veterans with at least one service or prescription provided by or paid for by VA during the year. Using this methodology, we estimated 3.6 million nonelderly VA patients during 2015, which is similar to the figure reported in the 2015 Survey of Veteran Enrollee's Health and Use of Health Care, VA's annual survey of veterans enrolled in VA health care (Gasper et al., 2015).

Following methods used in Eibner et al. (2015), we focused on counts of health care events rather than costs or spending (Appendix A). We focused on VA and total health care use over the period 2008–2014 in three categories: office-based visits, inpatient surgeries, and prescription drugs. We produced estimates separately for all nonelderly veterans (including ineligible or eligible but nonenrolled veterans) and for VA patients.

Table 3.3 summarizes patterns of VA and total health care utilization by reporting nonelderly veterans' per capita annual use of VA care and total health care. These data confirm that patterns of reliance documented in Eibner et al. (2015) broadly apply to nonelderly veterans, as well to as the overall veteran population: Most care provided to nonelderly veterans is rendered outside VA. A similar pattern is apparent even when we exclude ineligible and nonenrolled veterans from the sample by restricting attention to current VA patients: VA use accounts for less than half of care rendered to VA patients, while the average of individual-level reliance ranges between 40 and 55 percent for the three types of care we examined.

Table 3.3. Annual Health Care Use and VA Reliance by Nonelderly Veterans and VA Patients

	All Veterans			VA Patients		
Type of Care	Per Capita Annual VA Use	Per Capita Annual Total Use	Average Individual Reliance for Veterans Using Care	Per Capita Annual VA Use	Per Capita Annual Total Use	Average Individual Reliance for VA Patients Using Care
Office-based visits	1.1	5.5	21.2%	3.6	8.7	54.6%
Inpatient surgery	0.016	0.050	30.8%	0.052	0.113	46.9%
Prescription drugs	3.1	14.3	15.9%	10.0	23.9	40.3%

SOURCE: Authors' calculations, 2008–2014 MEPS Household Component full-year consolidated files and selected event files.
NOTES: This table reports unadjusted average VA and total use of selected health care services and prescription drugs for nonelderly veterans over the period 2008–2014. Use estimates are reported as annual counts of health care events (numbers of office visits, surgeries, or prescriptions filled) per capita. Average individual reliance is the average of individual-level reliance for veterans using any health services and thus represents the average percentage of care received from VA by those receiving care; individual-level reliance is not defined for individuals who receive no care in a given category, which can lead to differences between average reliance and the ratio between per capita VA use and per capita total use.

Nonelderly VA Patients Without Another Source of Insurance Coverage Rely More on VA for Health Care Than VA Patients Who Have Another Source of Coverage Do

Because most veterans are covered by non-VA health insurance even if they are enrolled in VA, changes in veterans' non-VA health insurance status are likely to affect the level of demand for VA care. For example, a VA-enrolled veteran who loses non-VA health insurance will likely increase reliance on VA for health care. In addition to increasing demand for VA services, it is possible that veterans losing insurance might reduce the total volume of health care they consume if not all of the care they would have consumed outside VA can be easily replaced with VA care.

To describe the cross-sectional association between non-VA insurance status and use of VA care, Table 3.4 reports regression-adjusted VA and total health care use for nonelderly veterans, stratified by insurance status. Nonelderly VA patients who lack non-VA insurance use VA at significantly higher rates for office-based visits (1.1 additional visits per year, or 35 percent more) and prescription drugs (2.86 additional prescriptions per year, or 43 percent more). Veterans without non-VA insurance may use slightly less total care (from all payers and sources) in these categories, but differences in total care are not significant. Adjusted rates of inpatient surgery receipt from VA are not associated with non-VA insurance status, but VA patients who lack non-VA insurance use significantly less inpatient surgery overall (0.039 fewer surgeries per year, or 49 percent less). Across all three categories of care, adjusted VA reliance is substantially higher for VA patients who lack non-VA insurance.

Table 3.4. VA and Total Health Care Use and VA Reliance for Nonelderly VA Patients, by Non-VA Health Insurance Status

	With Non-VA Insurance	Without Non-VA Insurance	Difference (Insured Minus Uninsured)
Office-based visits			
Adjusted VA use (annual visits per capita)	3.10	4.20	−1.10***
Adjusted all-payer use (annual visits per capita)	8.34	7.35	0.99
Adjusted VA reliance	37%	57%	−20%***
Inpatient surgery			
Adjusted VA use (annual surgeries per capita)	0.033	0.029	0.004
Adjusted all-payer use (annual surgeries per capita)	0.080	0.041	0.039**
Adjusted VA reliance	41%	71%	−30%***
Prescription drugs			
Adjusted VA use (annual prescriptions per capita)	6.64	9.50	−2.86**
Adjusted all-payer use (annual prescriptions per capita)	20.12	18.71	1.41
Adjusted VA reliance	33%	51%	−18%***

SOURCE: Authors' calculations, 2008–2014 MEPS.
NOTES: The sample was restricted to nonelderly VA patients. VA and total use were adjusted for age, family income, self-reported health, race/ethnicity, and year using Poisson regression. Adjusted reliance was calculated as the ratio of adjusted VA use to adjusted total use. Full regression coefficients are reported in Appendix A.
* $p < 0.10$, ** $p < 0.05$, *** $p < 0.01$. The significance of differences in use is based on Poisson regression coefficients. The significance of differences in reliance is based on the Wald test for difference in adjusted reliance.

While the differences in Table 3.4 are adjusted for observable characteristics that affect demand for health care, these estimates should not be interpreted as capturing the *causal* effect of non-VA insurance on demand for VA health care. Much of the variation in insurance status that drives the patterns observed in the table is likely to reflect reverse causation from health status or VA eligibility to non-VA insurance enrollment decisions. Observational studies on the association between non-VA insurance and VA use might find that non-VA insurance is not associated with VA use (Yoon et al., 2017), a finding that is consistent with the pattern of inpatient surgery use reported in Table 3.4.

To analyze the effect of changes in insurance coverage on VA use, it is necessary to know the *causal* effect of non-VA insurance on VA use. By *causal effect*, we mean the change in VA use that would result from changing a veteran's non-VA insurance status while holding constant all other factors—both observable and unobservable—that affect health care use. Research that captures the causal effect of non-VA insurance on VA use is very limited, but there are two studies with credible research designs that provide evidence on this question. Only one of these studies directly estimates the causal effect of non-VA health insurance on VA enrollees' VA use while accounting for self-selection of veterans into non-VA health insurance (Shen et al., 2008). Shen et al. found that private insurance reduced nonelderly veterans' probability of using any VA care and that private insurance reduced VA costs and the probability of any VA use specifically for both inpatient and prescription drug utilization. Their estimates imply that the percentage changes in VA costs resulting from private insurance are comparable in magnitude to the adjusted differences reported in Table 3.4, with private insurance reducing total VA costs by 33.7 percent, reducing VA inpatient costs by 26.2 percent, and reducing prescription drug costs by 38.9 percent. Another study with a credible research design examined the causal effect of Medicaid eligibility on VA use but did not incorporate data on Medicaid enrollment or insurance coverage (Frakt, Hanchate, and Pizer, 2015). This study, which examined utilization data at the VA sector level and thus included nonenrolled veterans as well as enrollees, found strong evidence that Medicaid eligibility reduced VA outpatient and inpatient use; VA enrollment also fell as a result of expanded Medicaid eligibility. Frakt, Hanchate, and Pizer (2015) estimated that a 10-percent increase in Medicaid eligibility among nonelderly veterans (representing an increase of 0.89 percentage points in their sample) reduced VA enrollment by 1.1 percent, reduced VA inpatient days by 0.65 percent, and reduced outpatient clinic stops by 1.4 percent. Because most adults who gain Medicaid eligibility as a result of coverage expansions do not actually take up Medicaid coverage, these estimated effects of Medicaid *eligibility* suggest that the effect of Medicaid *enrollment* on VA demand may be quite large. We provide further discussion of the research literature on health insurance and nonelderly veterans' use of VA care in Appendix A.

In the case of ACA repeal, where the policy intervention under consideration is likely to reduce insurance, we would specifically like to know how the *loss* of health insurance coverage would affect VA utilization among individuals who would otherwise be insured. The effect of losing insurance might not be symmetric with the effect of gaining insurance for several reasons: Compared with uninsured individuals, those who have had insurance in the past may be more comfortable seeking out care, may be more likely to have received diagnoses that might increase use of care in the future, or may be more likely to be undergoing treatment that they might seek to continue at a different provider after losing insurance.

In an attempt to learn specifically about the effect of losing non-VA insurance on VA utilization, we identified a sample of veterans who gained or lost non-VA insurance while under observation in the MEPS. We did find suggestive evidence that veterans losing non-VA insurance substantially increased their demand for VA care (by 49 percent) after losing insurance, while veterans gaining non-VA insurance may have decreased their VA use. However, available samples in the MEPS were very limited, resulting in very imprecise estimates, and we did not find evidence of similar relationships for inpatient surgery or prescription drugs. Because the MEPS lacks a large-enough sample of nonelderly veterans who switch insurance status while under observation to enable precise estimation of how non-VA insurance affects health care use, we used estimates from the peer-reviewed research literature to predict the impact of ACA repeal (see the next chapter) rather than using estimates obtained from our analysis of the MEPS.

4. How Would ACA Repeal Proposals Affect Veterans' Insurance Coverage and Use of VA Health Care?

To assess the potential effect of ACA repeal on veterans' demand for and reliance on VA care, we developed a model to examine three scenarios (see Table 4.1).[11] Our first scenario models the effect of reversing the insurance coverage gains experienced between 2013 and 2015. Our second and third scenarios predict the effect of the AHCA at two points in the future: 2020 and 2026. Our modeling framework used estimates derived from the peer-reviewed literature to capture the effect of insurance status on veterans' use of VA and total health care. By combining these estimates with scenarios defining changes in insurance status for different subgroups of veterans, we were able to calculate how utilization would change relative to a baseline scenario under the coverage changes anticipated under different ACA repeal options. As we will discuss, our baseline is the level of VA care received by veterans in 2015, and so our analysis produces estimates of how coverage changes like those anticipated under ACA repeal would have affected veterans in 2015. Forecasting changes in VA demand was beyond the scope of this study, since valid forecasts require a baseline that accounts for demographic change and trends in health status and health care needs.

---

[11] Technical details of this model and additional estimates are presented in Appendix A.

Table 4.1. ACA Repeal Scenarios

	Baseline Scenario	Reverse ACA Coverage Gains	AHCA, 2020 Provisions	AHCA, 2026 Provisions
Scenario description	Uninsurance rates and average VA and total use for eight age, income, and health status cells calculated for 2015 veteran population	Percentage change in uninsurance due to reversing coverage gains calculated using the ratio of the adjusted 2013 uninsurance rate to the adjusted 2015 uninsurance rate for groups of veterans defined by age and income	Percentage change in uninsurance due to AHCA coverage provisions calculated by reweighting COMPARE-augmented U.S. Census Bureau Survey of Income and Program Participation data to match the age, income, gender, and health status distribution of the 2015 nonelderly veteran population and calculating the percentage increase in uninsurance for age, income, and health status groups. 2020 AHCA coverage estimates are reported in Eibner, Liu, and Nowak (2017).	
Source of coverage changes	2015 ACS; 2015 NHIS	2013–2015 ACS	COMPARE	COMPARE
Key provisions modeled	N/A	This scenario does not explicitly model the ACA: All changes in coverage between 2013 and 2015 are reversed.	<ul><li>Age-dependent tax credits between \$2,000 and \$4,000</li><li>Age-rating bands widened to 5:1</li><li>Individual mandate eliminated</li><li>Employer mandate eliminated</li><li>Continuous coverage requirement established</li><li>Actuarial value requirements eliminated</li><li>Health savings accounts expanded</li><li>Excise tax on high-cost employer plans delayed until 2026</li><li>Patient and State Stability Fund established</li><li>Cost-sharing reductions eliminated</li><li>Medicaid expansion option eliminated in 2019; enhanced federal funding ends in 2019; beginning in 2020, federal funding converted from open-ended entitlement to per capita cap indexed to CPI-M for nondisabled populations and CPI-M plus 1 percentage point for aged, blind, and disabled populations</li></ul>	
Average percentage uninsured	5.8%	9.1%	9.6%	10.4%
Average percentage-point increase in uninsurance (relative to current law)	N/A	+3.3	+3.8	+4.6

NOTES: For all scenarios, the percentage-point change in coverage is calculated for eight age, income, and health status cells by applying percentage changes in uninsurance to the 2015 baseline uninsurance rate for each age, income, and health status cell as estimated in the 2015 NHIS. AHCA analysis based on bill as amended March 20, 2017 (U.S. Congress, 2017). CPI-M = Medical Consumer Price Index.

Our first scenario captures how demand for VA care in 2015 would have differed if the coverage gains experienced by veterans between 2013 and 2015 had not taken place. To do this, we specified a counterfactual in which the 2015 veteran population was covered by insurance at the rates observed in 2013 (after adjusting for individual characteristics). We then used the model described later in this chapter to analyze how much more VA care veterans in 2015 would have used at these lower rates of insurance coverage. As noted previously, sample sizes of nonelderly veterans in the 2014 MEPS were inadequate to estimate the impacts of the ACA with sufficient precision, so analysis of this scenario gives us a way to understand the changes that have followed ACA implementation. However, while we adjust our estimated coverage changes for demographics, we cannot disentangle the overall effect of the ACA from other time trends. This scenario also may not capture the effects of an ACA repeal that returned health policy to the 2013 status quo.[12] Even so, we believe that this scenario is useful as a hypothetical counterfactual that provides a point of reference for our analysis of the AHCA.

Our second scenario used predicted insurance coverage changes from RAND's COMPARE model to develop scenarios meant to illustrate how changes in insurance status anticipated under the AHCA (as amended March 20, 2017) might affect VA use and reliance. COMPARE is a microsimulation model that has been widely used to analyze how changes in federal health policy will affect the level and source of health insurance coverage across the U.S. population. The analysis we build on here, which was presented in Eibner, Liu, and Nowak (2017), modeled the AHCA's proposed changes to the Marketplaces, Medicaid, and other policy levers that affect insurance coverage; these provisions are listed in Table 4.1. Provisions modeled include elimination of the individual and employer mandates, imposition of a continuous coverage requirement, expanded health savings accounts, and delay of the excise tax on high-cost employer plans (i.e., the "Cadillac" tax). Marketplace provisions modeled include age-dependent tax credits, wider (5:1) age-rating bands, elimination of actuarial value requirements, elimination of cost-sharing reductions, and establishment of the Patient and State Stability Fund (which would provide up to $100 billion in reinsurance funding over 2018–2026). Medicaid provisions modeled included elimination of the Medicaid expansion option for states that had not expanded by 2019, as well as conversion of federal Medicaid contributions from an open-ended entitlement to a capped per capita allocation. The allocation would be indexed to CPI-M for nondisabled and nonelderly Medicaid enrollees and to CPI-M plus 1 percentage point for blind, elderly, and disabled enrollees.[13]

Eibner, Liu, and Nowak (2017) found that the AHCA would have reduced health insurance coverage by 14.0 million in 2020 and by 19.7 million in 2026, with the bulk of the coverage

---

[12] It is not clear whether the impacts on VA demand of a return to the pre-ACA status quo would be larger or smaller than indicated by this scenario. New Medicaid enrollees who were eligible but unenrolled prior to the ACA might remain insured even if the ACA were repealed, suggesting that a return to the pre-ACA status quo would not fully reverse the observed coverage gains. However, a similar form of inertia may apply to VA enrollment if new VA enrollees who enrolled because of ACA outreach efforts would continue to use VA care at higher rates than if the ACA had never taken effect.

[13] See Eibner, Liu, and Nowak (2017) for full estimates and additional details.

losses in both scenarios due to reduced Medicaid enrollment. COMPARE estimated smaller coverage losses than the CBO score of the AHCA in part because of differences in the methods used by COMPARE and CBO to model the performance of the individual market and employer decisions to continue offering employer-sponsored insurance under the AHCA; Medicaid coverage losses estimated by COMPARE are nearly identical to those estimated by CBO, however.[14]

Because COMPARE is not designed to provide estimates of health insurance coverage specific to veterans, we developed our AHCA scenario by dividing the COMPARE microsimulation output and the nonelderly veteran population into eight population cells defined by combinations of age (50 or older versus younger than 50), family income (at least 200 percent of FPL versus under 200 percent of the FPL), and self-reported health status (good or better versus fair or poor). We then reweighted the COMPARE microsimulation sample to match the 2015 veteran population distribution of age, gender, family income, and health status. The critical assumption is that coverage changes due to the AHCA would be similar for veterans and nonveterans who are identical in terms of age, gender, income, and health status. This assumption is not directly testable with respect to the AHCA, but we attempted to validate this assumption by comparing regression-adjusted coverage changes between 2013 and 2015 for veterans and nonveterans. There were some differences, but we found that proportional coverage changes for veterans in each population cell were within 10 to 20 percent of the changes predicted using data on nonveteran adults. We provide further details in Appendix A.

Predicted Effect of ACA Repeal Scenarios on Nonelderly Veterans' Insurance Coverage

The predicted effects of ACA repeal scenarios on nonelderly veterans' insurance coverage are illustrated in Figure 4.1. Several patterns are noteworthy. Reflecting the broad-based coverage gains that occurred after ACA implementation, reversal of these coverage gains leads to lower levels of non-VA insurance coverage for all demographic groups. By 2020, the AHCA would slightly increase non-VA coverage for higher-income young veterans but would result in loss of coverage similar to or slightly larger than the effects of simply reversing the ACA for all other groups. Loss of coverage for lower-income veterans age 50 and older would be substantially larger under the AHCA than under the reversal of ACA coverage gains, a fact that reflects the scope of Medicaid financing changes under the AHCA. Finally, 2026 coverage changes under the AHCA are larger for older veterans at all income levels, with the increased magnitude of coverage loss most likely reflecting the increasing effect of Medicaid financing changes. The concentration of coverage losses among older adults also is likely to reflect the AHCA's adoption of 5:1 age bands in concert with changes that decouple the value of premium subsidies from the price of coverage.

---

[14] See Eibner, Liu, and Nowak (2017) for full estimates and additional details.

Figure 4.1. Predicted Non-VA Uninsurance Changes Under ACA Repeal and Replace Scenarios, by Age, Family Income, and Health Status

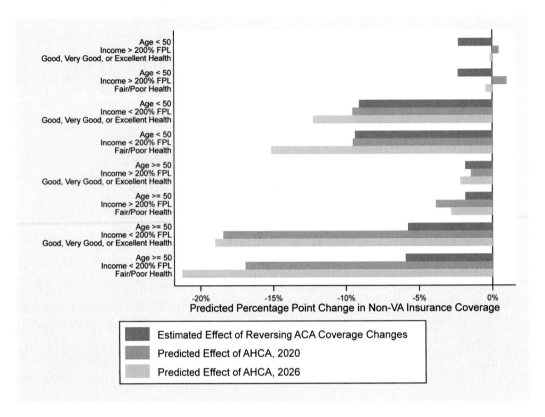

NOTES: This figure depicts scenario inputs used in analysis of ACA repeal, stratified by age, family income, and health status. Coverage changes under "Estimated Effect of Reversing ACA Coverage Changes" were derived from NHIS and ACS estimates of change in non-VA uninsurance between 2013 and 2015 stratified by age, income, and health status. "Predicted Effect of AHCA" was derived from 2015 ACS and NHIS estimates and RAND COMPARE analysis of the AHCA as amended March 20, 2017. See Appendix A for details.

Predicted Effect of ACA Repeal Scenarios on Nonelderly Veterans' Use of VA Health Care

We then estimated a statistical model using data from the 2008–2014 MEPS to capture how nonelderly veterans' use of VA and non-VA health care varies with their non-VA insurance status and their individual characteristics, including age, gender, race/ethnicity, family income, and health status. Combined with our scenarios, which specify how many veterans in each population cell would lose non-VA insurance, our statistical model gives us a way to calculate the level of VA use and reliance when covered by non-VA insurance for the average veteran who would lose coverage under the AHCA. The central assumption of this model is that non-VA insurance has a constant proportional effect on the use of VA and non-VA care, holding other factors constant.[15]

---

[15] This functional form assumption is standard in the analysis of health care utilization data, which is inherently nonnegative and skewed. Further details on model specification are presented in Appendix A.

As Figure 4.1 makes clear, coverage changes under either reversal of the ACA or implementation of the AHCA would vary widely across subgroups of veterans defined by age, income, and health status. The mix of veterans who lose insurance under a given scenario is the mechanism at the heart of our analysis of ACA repeal, since VA health care use and total health care use also vary systematically across these demographic groups. By assuming a constant proportional response of health care use to the loss of insurance, our model effectively assumes that a given increase in the uninsured population that is concentrated among veterans with high demand for health care will have a larger impact on the total volume of health care use than an equivalent increase in the uninsured population among healthy veterans who rarely use health care.

Figure 4.2 illustrates differences across these demographic groups in the share of nonelderly veterans who are VA patients. Low-income veterans in poor health are more likely than not to use VA care at least once in a year, while healthier and higher-income veterans are less likely to use any VA care. This pattern is in line with the eligibility rules used by VA. We show, in Appendix A, that VA use and VA reliance also tend to be higher for lower-income, older, and less-healthy veterans.

**Figure 4.2. Proportion of Veterans Using VA Care,
by Age, Income, and Health Status**

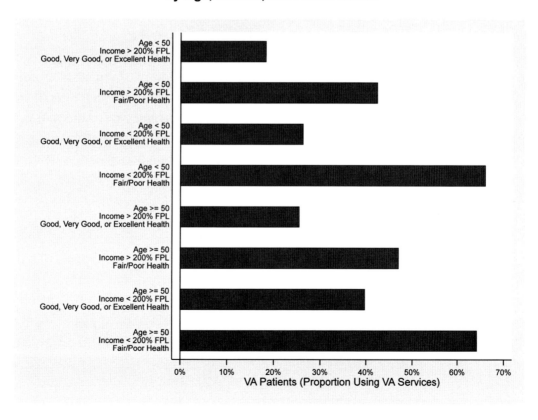

SOURCE: Authors' calculations, 2008–2014 MEPS.

The COMPARE analysis we drew on to develop our scenarios focused on the impacts of the AHCA in the years 2020 and 2026. To avoid the uncertainty and modeling complexity involved in forecasting the baseline demographic structure and insurance status of the nonelderly veteran population in these future years, all our analyses use actual data (from the ACS and NHIS) on the 2015 demographics, health status, and insurance status of nonelderly veterans to define the baseline scenario. Because we did not model anticipated demographic changes in the veteran population, our results should not be interpreted as forecasts of VA demand for future years. Rather, these estimates reflect how changes in patterns of insurance coverage proportional to those forecast under the AHCA would have affected VA and total health care use by the nonelderly veteran population in 2015. We also note that we did not explicitly model VA enrollment decisions, in large part because the MEPS does not measure VA coverage or VA enrollment. Instead, we modeled per capita VA use for the noninstitutionalized nonelderly veteran population, including nonenrolled and ineligible veterans as well as VA enrollees. We derived our parameters from a study that focused on VA enrollees (Shen et al., 2008), so our estimates will be valid if non-VA insurance does not affect VA enrollment. Prior research on this question yielded mixed results (Frakt, Hanchate, and Pizer, 2015; Wong et al., 2014; Chan et al., 2014), and we did not find strong evidence that the Medicaid expansion affected VA enrollment; some estimates suggested that Medicaid expansion reduced VA enrollment, but these were not statistically significant. In the event that future coverage losses increase VA enrollment, our estimates of changes in VA use may understate actual changes.

The critical inputs to our analysis are parameters capturing the percentage change in VA use and overall health care use resulting from a change from insurance to uninsurance. Because we are interested in the impact of a policy change that would modify health insurance status but leave other individual characteristics constant, the ideal source for identifying these parameters would be a randomized controlled trial. No such experimental estimates exist for the causal effect of non-VA insurance on use of VA care, so we instead chose parameters after a review of peer-reviewed studies that estimated the effect of non-VA insurance on nonelderly veterans' VA use with appropriate research designs for causal inference (Frakt, Hanchate, and Pizer, 2015; Shen et al., 2008). We drew our central parameters from Shen et al. (2008) because the authors were able to estimate the effect of insurance coverage on VA use, whereas Frakt, Hanchate, and Pizer (2015) did not directly observe insurance status and instead modeled the effect of expansions in Medicaid eligibility for nonelderly adults. Both of these studies indicate that non-VA insurance reduces use of VA care, with the study by Frakt, Hanchate, and Pizer (2015) suggesting that changes in insurance coverage have somewhat larger effects on VA demand than estimated by Shen et al. (2008). We discuss these studies in greater detail in Appendix A. For the effect of non-VA uninsurance on overall health care use, we derived estimates from the results of the Oregon Health Study, which is a large-scale randomized study measuring the effect of Medicaid coverage (relative to uninsurance) on health care utilization and other outcomes (Baicker et al., 2013; Finkelstein et al., 2012).

In our central analysis, we assumed that the loss of non-VA health insurance would increase a nonelderly veteran's VA use by 33.7 percent for office-based visits, by 26.2 percent for inpatient surgery, and by 38.9 percent for prescription drugs; we also assumed that loss of non-

VA insurance would reduce a veteran's total health care use by 32.9 percent for office-based visits, by 25.9 percent for inpatient surgery, and by 26.8 percent for prescription drugs. The percentage changes in inpatient and prescription drug VA use are the changes in VA costs for those services implied by the Shen et al. (2008) estimates of the effect of private insurance on VA use among enrollees. For office-based visits, we used the Shen et al. estimate for total VA spending. While the association between insurance coverage and VA use documented in Table 3.4 does not reflect a causal relationship, the differences in office-based and prescription drug use reported in that table are similar in magnitude to the effects implied by Shen et al. While it would be ideal to have a separate set of parameters for the loss of Medicaid coverage, the causal effects of Medicaid eligibility reported by Frakt, Hanchate, and Pizer (2015) imply changes in VA use that are as large or larger than our elasticities. Our estimates of changes in VA use after veterans lost insurance also suggest that larger increases in VA use of office-based visits might be possible. We accordingly view the Shen et al. estimates as reasonable or slightly conservative estimates of the effect of non-VA insurance on VA use. To reflect the uncertainty inherent in these assumptions, we conducted sensitivity analyses under alternative values of all parameters. Additional details on our assumptions about the effect of insurance on health care use and the results of our sensitivity analyses are presented in Appendix A.

Reversal of Post-ACA Coverage Gains Would Increase Nonelderly Veterans' Use of VA Health Care; Coverage Changes Anticipated Under the AHCA Would Have Even Larger Impacts

We estimated that ACA repeal would increase veterans' demand for and reliance on VA health care while reducing the total amount of health care received by this population (Table 4.2). Because estimates of the causal effect of insurance on VA demand suggest that demand for office-based visits, inpatient surgery, and prescription drugs all have broadly similar responses to the loss of non-VA insurance, the percentage changes in VA demand are similar in magnitude for all three types of care within each scenario.

Our first scenario, which involves reversing the coverage gains that occurred between 2013 and 2015, would increase the number of VA office visits by nonelderly veterans by 1.2 percent, the number of VA inpatient surgeries by 1.0 percent, and the number of VA prescriptions dispensed by 1.3 percent. Despite increases in VA health care use, overall health care use (from any source) by nonelderly veterans would fall by 0.8 to 1.0 percent in each of these categories. Average VA reliance would increase by 0.20 to 0.37 percentage points. These estimates represent our best nationwide estimate of changes in nonelderly veterans' use of VA and non-VA health care since the ACA's major coverage expansions took effect, as publicly available data sources do not yet contain sufficient post-ACA data to obtain precise estimates of the ACA's effect on VA and non-VA use for nonelderly veterans. However, as noted previously, coverage changes between 2013 and 2015 may not be fully attributable to the ACA.

Table 4.2. Predicted Change in VA Use and Reliance Due to ACA Repeal

		Change from Baseline		
Office-Based Visits	**2015 Baseline**	**Reverse ACA Coverage Changes**	**AHCA (2020)**	**AHCA (2026)**
VA visits	10,698,205	+124,985	+207,478	+243,384
(percentage change)		+1.17%	+1.94%	+2.28%
All-payer visits	56,169,585	−557,721	−811,702	−939,353
(percentage change)		−0.99%	−1.45%	−1.67%
Reliance	19.05%	19.46%	19.70%	19.81%
(change in percentage points)		+0.24%	+0.47%	+0.59%
Inpatient Surgery				
VA surgeries	157,579	+1,531	+3,047	+3,525
(percentage change)		+0.97%	+1.93%	+2.24%
All-payer surgeries	528,851	−4,468	−8,244	−9,310
(percentage change)		−0.84%	−1.56%	−1.76%
Reliance	29.80%	30.34%	30.85%	31.01%
(change in percentage points)		+0.37%	+0.88%	+1.04%
Prescription Drugs				
VA prescriptions	28,410,071	+376,659	+798,551	+911,238
(percentage change)		+1.33%	+2.81%	+3.21%
All-payer prescriptions	145,225,712	−1,210,961	−2,171,561	−2,444,801
(percentage change)		−0.83%	−1.50%	−1.68%
Reliance	19.56%	19.99%	20.42%	20.54%
(change in percentage points)		+0.20%	+0.63%	+0.75%

NOTE: See Appendix A for details.

Our second and third scenarios, which model the effects of the AHCA in 2020 and 2026, predict larger shifts in VA and total health care use than would result from simply reversing the coverage gains that occurred after the ACA went into effect. The changes in utilization predicted under the AHCA provisions in effect by 2026, holding the veteran population constant, are significant. If the AHCA provisions had been in effect in 2015, we estimated that the quantity of care provided by VA would have been higher by roughly 245,000 office-based visits (a 2.3-percent increase), 3,500 inpatient surgeries (a 2.2-percent increase), and 910,000 prescriptions (a 3.2-percent increase). These increases are several times larger than those that would have resulted from simply reversing the coverage gains that occurred after ACA implementation.

The difference between the effects of the AHCA and the effects of reversing the 2013–2015 coverage gains is driven in large part by the demographic composition of the population at risk of losing coverage under the AHCA. As summarized in Table 4.1, the overall coverage change under the AHCA in 2020 is only 15 percent (0.5 percentage points) larger than the change between 2013 and 2015. However, this moderate difference in average coverage changes masks more-dramatic differences in terms of how coverage losses are allocated across groups of veterans. Under the AHCA, COMPARE predicts slightly higher coverage for young, high-income veterans, but these gains are offset by much sharper coverage losses for lower-income, less-healthy, and older veterans. The latter groups of veterans have higher VA use, and so reductions in their rates of coverage have a disproportionate effect on VA demand: While the number of veterans losing insurance under the AHCA's 2020 provisions is only 15 percent larger than the number losing insurance from reversal of the ACA's coverage gains, the increase in VA demand resulting from this loss of coverage is 65 to 100 percent larger.

Higher coverage losses under the AHCA's 2026 provisions and their skew toward lower-income veterans reflect the compounding effect of Medicaid changes as the per capita financing approach proposed in the AHCA ratchets down spending relative to current law. To some extent, the concentration of coverage losses among older adults also is likely to reflect the AHCA's adoption of 5:1 age bands in concert with changes that decouple the value of premium subsidies from the price of coverage.

The impact on VA care of the AHCA's 2026 provisions is thus larger than under the other scenarios for two key reasons. First, overall reductions of insurance in 2026 are greater than those due to reversing the ACA's coverage gains or the AHCA in 2020. Second, reductions in coverage are more sharply skewed toward veterans with low family incomes and those in poor health. As illustrated by Figure 4.2, low-income veterans in fair or poor health are most likely to be VA patients, due both to their high overall health care needs and to the fact that VA eligibility incorporates both economic need and health status, among other factors. Finally, a slight reduction in non-VA coverage (between 1.6 and 1.9 percentage points more uninsured veterans) among higher-income veterans ages 50–64 also contributed to the decrease in VA demand. Higher-income veterans ages 50–64 accounted for two in five nonelderly veterans in 2015, and so slight reductions in insurance coverage for these groups can have larger implications for overall VA demand than one might conclude from looking at the incremental change in insurance status in isolation.

Table 4.2 also reports changes in total health care use that would result under the three scenarios we analyzed. The estimates we use to predict changes in total health care use are more similar across types of care than those we used to analyze VA use, and so the proportional reductions in total health care use resulting from ACA repeal are also similar across types of service. Total health care use would have been around 0.8 to 1.0 percent lower if the ACA's coverage gains were reversed, 1.2 to 1.4 percent lower under the coverage changes predicted to result from the AHCA's 2020 provisions, and 1.7 to 1.8 percent lower under the coverage changes predicted to result from the AHCA's 2026 provisions. VA reliance would accordingly have increased by between 0.77 and 1.22 percentage points under the AHCA's 2026 provisions.

This analysis has a number of important limitations that should be noted when interpreting our results. As noted previously, our central assumptions about the response of VA and total health care use to loss of insurance might not hold in practice. In particular, we relied on estimates developed for the national population (including nonveterans) to define our AHCA scenario, and we likewise used parameters drawn from a study that did not focus specifically on the veteran population. Similarly, our key parameters from VA were estimated for a sample of nonelderly veterans collected nearly two decades ago, and so one might raise concerns about their validity for today's health system and veteran population. In large part, these limitations reflect the relative scarcity of carefully designed empirical studies on the causal relationship between non-VA insurance status and VA use. We believe that reweighting COMPARE to match the veteran population should make it more credible to use COMPARE estimates in our analysis. The behavioral responses to insurance captured in the Shen et al. estimates are corroborated by Frakt, Hanchate, and Pizer (2015), who use more-recent data from 2002–2008.

Although we have firmer empirical support for our total health care elasticities (because they are derived from the gold-standard, experimental Oregon Health Study), one might also worry about the external validity of the Oregon Health Study elasticities for our setting.[16] The key concern is that uninsured subjects in the Oregon Health Study likely had more-limited access to care than do uninsured VA enrollees, suggesting that the effect of non-VA uninsurance on total use of health care might be smaller in magnitude (i.e., less negative) for VA enrollees than suggested by the results of the Oregon Heath Study. This would affect our estimates of changes in total health care use and reliance but not our estimates of VA demand.

That said, there are also reasons to think that the Oregon Health Study would have strong external validity for the population of veterans most likely to lose health insurance under ACA repeal or a reform similar to the AHCA. The Oregon Health Study estimates the effect of Medicaid coverage on low-income, nondisabled adults; to the extent that the coverage impacts of the AHCA or other reforms are concentrated among low-income adults and Medicaid enrollees, we might expect to see similar effects to those observed in Oregon. In addition, the Oregon

---

[16] Care provided at VA hospitals was not captured in the Oregon Health Study, so the inclusion of VA-eligible veterans in the sample might have biased the effects of the study downward as an estimate of total use. It is unlikely, however, that any of the Oregon Health Study subjects were VA-eligible because the population in the study consisted of low-income adults who had been uninsured for six months or more but had applied for Oregon's Medicaid state plan.

Health Study subjects had certain demographic and medical characteristics that made the subjects more comparable to veterans than a nationally representative sample would have been. Compared with the overall U.S. population, the Oregon study subjects were older and less likely to be nonwhite. In addition, both Oregon study subjects and nonelderly veterans were more likely to have chronic health conditions than the general nonelderly population. However, there are also important differences, such as the proportion who are female, between the two populations. It is not clear how these compositional differences might affect the validity of the Oregon study estimates for our setting.

To assess the robustness of our analysis to uncertainty about the effect of uninsurance on health care use, we conducted sensitivity analyses meant to indicate the range of uncertainty about the effect of ACA repeal on VA use and reliance. We defined a "low-reliance" simulation in which we reduced the VA use parameters by half and doubled the total health care use parameters, and we defined a "high-reliance" scenario in which we doubled the VA use parameters and reduced the total health care use parameters by half. These sensitivity analyses naturally led to a wide range for changes in VA use and reliance. For example, the estimated 3.2-percent increase in prescriptions that we predicted under the 2026 provisions of the AHCA scenario might range from a 1.5-percent increase under the low-reliance assumptions to a 7.7-percent increase under high-reliance assumptions, while the estimated increase in average reliance might range from 0.47 to 2.13 percentage points.

In Appendix A, we provide a more-extensive discussion of the evidence base on the response of VA demand to uninsurance. We note that there are several reasons to believe that our central parameter assumptions, as well as certain aspects of our modeling strategy, would tend to produce conservative estimates (in the sense of predicting smaller increases in VA use than might be likely). One factor is that we assume that—contrary to intuition—loss of insurance does not induce additional VA enrollment. We reviewed the empirical evidence on this question, including our own estimates of the ACA Medicaid expansion's effect, and did not find the evidence to point clearly to an answer to this question. This assumption may lead us to underestimate increases in VA demand if there is an enrollment response, as suggested by at least one highly credible study on this question (Frakt, Hanchate, and Pizer, 2015). In addition, the study on non-VA uninsurance and VA use that we consider to have the strongest quasi-experimental design also suggests strongly that the effect of non-VA uninsurance on VA use could be much higher than we have assumed here (Frakt, Hanchate, and Pizer, 2015). In this case, we suspect that deviations of VA use from our predictions would fall between our central assumptions and the larger increases found under our high-reliance assumptions. However, we emphasize that there is considerable uncertainty around our parameter assumptions and future changes in uninsurance and, accordingly, chose to take estimates directly from the research literature for our central assumptions.

State-Specific Impacts of ACA Repeal on VA Demand Will Depend on the Extent of Coverage Loss and the Age Structure of the State's Veteran Population

We also adapted a simplified version of our repeal model to produce state-specific estimates of the change in VA use that might be anticipated under the AHCA. These estimates are included in a separate Excel spreadsheet (available online at www.rand.org/t/RR1955) and are described more fully in Appendix B. The key insight behind these state-specific estimates is that states vary in both their exposure to ACA repeal and the age structure of their veteran populations. For example, New Jersey's veteran population is about 40 percent nonelderly, while Virginia's is about 60 percent nonelderly. A given change in VA use driven by insurance loss among the nonelderly population would hit Virginia harder than New Jersey. However, since Virginia has not yet implemented the ACA's Medicaid expansion, we might expect coverage losses among the nonelderly to be smaller in Virginia. Our state-specific estimates provide a way for states to assess which of these factors might dominate and thus gauge the shift in demand for VA care resulting from repeal.

Variation in our state-specific estimates derives largely from three dimensions of cross-state differences: Medicaid expansion status, the age structure of the veteran population under age 65, and the proportion of elderly versus nonelderly veterans. Because there is wide variation in the age structure of the veteran population across states, it may be important for VA planning to note that states with more nonelderly veterans and that have experienced greater coverage gains due to the ACA are likely to experience greater proportional increases in VA demand under current ACA repeal proposals. An important caveat to this conclusion is that we have not modeled changes in insurance status or VA use for the elderly or institutionalized veteran populations. Because changes to Medicaid financing proposed in both the AHCA and the BCRA would lead to reduced federal contributions for aged and disabled Medicaid beneficiaries, this omission could be important. Data sources other than the MEPS (such as the Health and Retirement Study or the National Health and Aging Trends Study) may be more appropriate for modeling these populations.

Other Consequences of ACA Repeal Are Harder to Quantify but May Be Important for Veterans and VA

The analysis of the AHCA presented in this chapter was based on estimates from RAND's COMPARE model so that we could use custom tabulations of the COMPARE model output to develop our scenario for veterans' insurance coverage. While the COMPARE estimates account in great detail for the AHCA's proposed changes to premium subsidies and Medicaid financing, key provisions of the AHCA and the BCRA pertaining to insurance regulation were not included in those COMPARE estimates. This modeling choice by the COMPARE research team reflects uncertainty about how states will use the expanded waiver authority offered under the AHCA and expanded under the BCRA. In this section, we highlight some of these provisions and provide a qualitative discussion of their potential impact on veterans and VA, as compared with the nonveteran population.

One in Three Nonelderly Veterans Has a Declinable Preexisting Condition

The AHCA allows states the option of requesting a waiver from a requirement that insurance policies offer coverage to all individuals, regardless of health status. Individual underwriting under the AHCA thus could apply to individuals who have a gap in coverage. Although it is not

43

known how many states would request such a waiver, removal of protections for individuals with preexisting health care conditions could affect a significant number of veterans. Using an algorithm developed by the Kaiser Family Foundation (Claxton et al., 2016), we estimated using the 2015 NHIS that one in three (34.5 percent, 95-percent confidence interval [31.2 percent, 37.8 percent]) nonelderly veterans had a health condition that would have made them uninsurable in the nongroup market under underwriting standards that prevailed prior to implementation of the ACA's reforms to insurance rating in 2014.[17]

Nonelderly veterans are more likely to have a declinable preexisting condition than other nonelderly adults in large part because veterans are older (by seven years) on average. Even after adjusting for age and gender, nonelderly veterans are 4.5 percentage points more likely to have a declinable preexisting condition than demographically comparable nonveterans.

Compared with other veterans, those with declinable preexisting conditions are older: 69 percent of nonelderly veterans with preexisting conditions are age 50 or over, compared with 40 percent of those without preexisting conditions. While we did not detect significant differences in the probability of uninsurance between veterans with and without preexisting conditions, there were systematic differences between these groups in the sources of non-VA insurance coverage: Veterans with preexisting conditions were more likely to be covered by Medicaid than veterans without preexisting conditions were (9.9 percent compared with 5.4 percent) and less likely to be covered by employer insurance (43.0 percent compared with 54.4 percent). This pattern suggests that nonelderly veterans with preexisting conditions may be more exposed to reductions in Medicaid eligibility than nonelderly veterans without preexisting conditions.

Less-Generous Insurance Plans May Reduce Affordability of Non-VA Care and Affect VA Demand

Our analysis of ACA repeal has been limited to changes in the number of uninsured nonelderly veterans that might result from current legislative proposals. Changes in the *quality* of insurance purchased by those who remain covered could also have substantial implications for veterans' access to care and demand for VA care. These changes are not modeled here because we lack information about precisely how states would use their waiver authority, and because we are aware of no rigorous evidence on the degree to which insured nonelderly veterans would substitute VA care for non-VA care in response to changes in the generosity of non-VA insurance (such as exclusions, policy limits, or higher deductibles).

Both the AHCA and the BCRA make a number of changes to insurance regulations that have the potential to make insurance coverage less generous. Reductions in the value of premium subsidies for many individual-market consumers would tend to incentivize selection of individual-market policies with higher deductibles. The use of states' waiver authority to modify the essential health benefits package is likely to adversely affect coverage for certain high-cost services in individual and small-group insurance plans.

---

[17] See Appendix A for details.

More subtly, there is some potential for expanded waiver authority to undermine consumer protections established by the ACA for large-employer plans, including the requirement that plans have an out-of-pocket maximum and the prohibition against annual and lifetime limits. This is because, under the ACA, these consumer protections apply to services defined as essential health benefits. Although CBO predicted that waivers would have little impact on whether high-cost services are *covered* by large employer plans (CBO, 2017b), an analysis by the Brookings Institution (Fiedler, 2017) argued that at least some large employers would be likely to reinstate policy limits and raise or eliminate out-of-pocket maximums for some high-cost services currently included in the essential health benefits. While there is some ambiguity in how the waivers in the AHCA would affect large employer plans, any possibility of changes to benefit design in employer-sponsored plans is noteworthy because employer-sponsored insurance is the predominant source of coverage for nonelderly adults.

While the ultimate impact of changes to the essential health benefits would depend on employer and insurer behavior, differences in the cost of and demand for different types of services makes it possible to predict which types of care are most likely to be affected. In its June 26, 2017, score of the BCRA, CBO predicted the following as a likely outcome of the bill's waiver provisions:

> Because a large portion of the population affected by additional waivers would be in states that narrow the scope of the [essential health benefits], CBO and [the Joint Committee on Taxation] expect insurance covering certain services to become more expensive—in some cases, extremely expensive. For example, if the [essential health benefits] were modified to drop coverage of services that have high costs and are used by few people, coverage for maternity care, mental health care, rehabilitative and habilitative treatment, and certain very expensive drugs could be at risk. (CBO, 2017b)

Anticipated reductions in the availability of maternity coverage might have limited impacts on the overwhelmingly male veteran population. Other changes to benefits, however, would seem to have the potential for major impacts on VA in light of the veteran population's unique health care needs. Previous RAND research has estimated that veterans of all ages have a higher age-adjusted prevalence of functional limitations, cancer, and mental health conditions than the nonveteran population (Eibner et al., 2015). Reliance on VA for high-cost specialty drugs might also be sensitive to the design of non-VA insurance plans. Research quantifying how non-VA insurance generosity affects VA demand is needed to assess these impacts, however, and thus warrants more attention from VA and independent researchers.

5. Discussion and Conclusions

Compared with other nonelderly adults, veterans are distinguished both by their unique health care needs and by their access to VA care. While VA helps to ensure that veterans are less likely to be uninsured than similar nonveterans, not all veterans are eligible for VA care, and nearly one in ten nonelderly veterans lacked any insurance or VA coverage in 2013.

After implementation of the ACA, the proportion of nonelderly veterans lacking any health coverage fell sharply due to increases in both Medicaid coverage and private coverage, including direct-purchase coverage obtained through the ACA Marketplaces. Comparison of similar veterans in expansion and nonexpansion states further suggests that the Medicaid expansion played an important role in raising insurance coverage rates. Of particular note is our finding that the Medicaid expansion led to larger increases in coverage among veterans living far from VA facilities. The higher take-up of Medicaid coverage by veterans living far from VA facilities suggests that the Medicaid expansion may have provided a valuable new coverage option to these veterans.

In addition to providing coverage to veterans who lacked any form of insurance, the ACA reduced the number of veterans who were enrolled in VA health care with no other source of coverage. Increases in dual VA and non-VA coverage, particularly VA coverage with Medicaid, were especially pronounced for disabled and low-income veterans. By increasing access to non-VA care, the ACA had the potential to reduce demands on the VA system and veterans' reliance on VA. The estimates reported in Table 4.2 suggest that the coverage changes that followed the ACA's implementation most likely led to modest reductions of 1.0 to 1.3 percent in nationwide VA demand, accounting for about 125,000 fewer office visits, 1,500 fewer surgeries, and 375,000 fewer prescriptions. We reiterate that these estimates do not account for other concurrent VA policy changes and other factors that may also have affected utilization; these additional factors should be taken into account when interpreting changes in total VA use over this period.

Our analysis of the coverage changes that might result from the AHCA highlights several findings that are likely applicable to any reform package with similar impacts on the uninsurance rates of different population groups. Specifically, we predict that the AHCA would lead to an increase in the number and proportion of nonelderly veterans without health insurance. We predict disproportionately large coverage losses among older, lower-income, and less-healthy nonelderly veterans. These veterans are more likely to be eligible for VA health care, and, as a result, we predict a significant increase in VA health care use, on the order of 260,000 additional office-based visits each year. Increases in demand for inpatient surgery and prescription drugs would likely be similar as a proportion of the relevant baselines. The effects of the AHCA on veterans' insurance status and use of health care exceed the effects of simply reversing post-ACA coverage changes, in part because the mix of veterans experiencing coverage changes is different and in part because the AHCA would lead to reductions in coverage larger than the gains we found after the ACA went into effect.

To some extent, the fact that coverage reductions are likely to be concentrated among older and less-healthy nonelderly veterans may be inherent in any bill that, like the AHCA, seeks to substantially reduce spending on Medicaid care or premium subsidies. While we did not have comparable cost data for VA and non-VA care that would allow us to assess the implications of the AHCA for VA budgets or total health care spending, the estimates we obtained on the long-term effects of the AHCA on VA use suggest that direct federal budgetary savings from the AHCA or similar bills may be slightly offset by increased VA demand among those veterans who lose their non-VA coverage.

Limitations

This analysis was limited in scope on several dimensions, as noted previously. Our use of self-reported survey data makes our estimates potentially subject to measurement error driven by respondent misreporting of the source of insurance. This is a known limitation of the ACS. Where possible, we corroborated our ACS estimates with data from the NHIS, in which the source of insurance is measured more accurately. However, it was not possible to reproduce estimates requiring state codes (such as our estimates of the Medicaid expansion's effects) with the public-use NHIS. Similarly, our imputed measure of priority group is likely subject to some classification errors at the individual level because we used a series of actuarial adjustments to match priority-group figures published by VA.

We also reiterate the difficulties inherent in using survey data to identify the veteran population and measure their involvement with VA. Discrepancies between the veteran populations identified in the ACS and NHIS (all veterans) and the MEPS (honorably discharged veterans) could mean that our MEPS estimates of per capita VA use for all veterans overstate VA use because dishonorably discharged veterans, who were ineligible for VA care at the time when our data were collected, are not included in our analysis of the MEPS. On the other hand, total volumes of VA inpatient stays and prescription drugs estimated in the MEPS are lower than administrative counts reported in VA budget requests. To the extent that the dishonorably discharged population is relatively small, the impact of any discrepancies on our overall estimates may be limited. In addition, the concept of *VA coverage* captured by the ACS bears an uncertain relationship to the concepts of VA enrollment and VA patient status. We have argued that individuals reporting VA coverage in the ACS most plausibly correspond to current VA patients, but this cannot be verified, and so caution is warranted in interpreting our VA coverage estimates.

The ACA and current legislative proposals to repeal and replace the ACA are large, complex pieces of legislation, and we were not able to address all the components of the AHCA in our quantitative analysis. In particular, we did not model changes in insurance design (such as higher deductibles) that seem likely under both the AHCA and the BCRA. CBO, in its analysis of the BCRA, predicts that higher deductibles in Marketplace plans would further discourage insurance purchases by low-income adults (CBO, 2017b). We also hypothesize that less-generous insurance policies would tend to increase VA reliance among veterans with non-VA insurance coverage, but this question has not been examined empirically by existing research. Our estimates of the AHCA, in short, do not capture all of the law's potential effects on nonelderly veterans. Furthermore, the extraordinary fluidity of the current political situation surrounding the AHCA and the BCRA means that the applicability of our estimates to future versions of these bills will depend on the extent to which patterns of coverage changes approximate or diverge from those anticipated under the AHCA. Despite this limitation, the broad similarities between the major coverage provisions of the AHCA and the BCRA suggest that our findings are likely to provide at least some useful guidance as to how these proposals might affect veterans and VA. The CBO scores of the AHCA and the BCRA predicted similarly sized reductions in health insurance coverage by 2026 relative to current law. As with the AHCA, reductions in insurance coverage under the BCRA are predicted to be largest for low-income adults, due to changes in federal Medicaid financing and changes to the Marketplaces that would make insurance less attractive to low-income and older adults (CBO, 2017b).

Any analysis like this by necessity assumes that there are no other policy changes happening that affect the outcomes of interest. Of course, this is never the case. For example, as the ACA was implemented, the Veterans Choice Act was also being rolled out, which increased VA-enrolled veterans' options for receiving VA care in their communities. Similarly, as ACA repeal legislation was introduced, legislation expanding the Choice program to additional VA-enrolled veterans was also being debated. Increasing access to VA community care for enrolled veterans will likely reduce demand for VA health care, which may modify any changes to VA demand as a result of ACA implementation or ACA repeal. Simultaneously, the veteran population itself is shrinking in size and changing in composition, which will affect VA demand both in the near and long term.

This changing VA environment complicates analysis of the effects of the ACA on VA health care. For example, between 2013 and 2015, VA coverage rates increased. In light of previous trends, it is very possible that coverage would have increased even more without the ACA, so the overall ACA effect may have been negative. Continuing growth of VA's community-care program, making VA care more accessible, may blunt the effects on veterans' health care access of any rollback in the ACA. This is particularly true with respect to Medicaid because any veteran eligible for Medicaid automatically qualifies for VA care. So far, the Trump administration appears ready to continue past efforts to make VA care more accessible. Existing data do not support analyzing these persistent trends in VA demand and controlling for them in analyses of the effects of the ACA on veterans.

Finally, our analysis was limited to nonelderly veterans; we did not analyze the potential impact of reduced federal Medicaid contributions on elderly veterans. In particular, the limits on federal Medicaid contributions specified in the AHCA may adversely affect coverage for elderly veterans in long-term care facilities and those eligible for full Medicaid benefits or who are dually enrolled in Medicare and Medicaid (Jacobson, Neuman, and Musumeci, 2017; Mann and Orris, 2017).

Conclusion

This report sought to analyze how veterans' insurance coverage has changed since the ACA went into effect, to characterize nonelderly veterans' use of VA and non-VA health care, and to provide insight into how current legislative proposals to repeal and replace the ACA might affect veterans' use of health care and demands on VA. We found that repeal and replacement of the ACA along lines similar to the AHCA would reduce the proportion of nonelderly veterans with insurance coverage outside VA. These coverage reductions would be concentrated among veterans who are lower income, older, and in worse health. Because the groups of veterans most likely to lose non-VA insurance coverage under these proposals also use VA services at higher rates, the potential impact of the AHCA or similar reforms on VA demand is likely to be larger than one might anticipate on the basis of information about overall average rates of VA use.

At the time this report was finalized (August 2017), the Senate and White House were debating the path forward for ACA repeal, and the short-term future of efforts to roll back the ACA's coverage expansions thus remained unclear. Even so, the findings of our analysis provide valuable information on the interaction between veterans' access to non-VA health insurance and their use of VA care. The estimates reported here will thus provide a useful starting point for understanding how veterans would fare under future proposals involving similar changes to the individual market or major reductions in federal Medicaid contributions. As the debate over the federal role in health insurance continues, a better understanding of the ways in which health insurance and health policy changes outside VA affect veterans' health care utilization is essential for VA and Congress to set health policy in a way that avoids creating unintended consequences for veterans or VA.

References

Baicker, Katherine, Sarah L. Taubman, Heidi L. Allen, Mira Bernstein, Jonathan H. Gruber, Joseph P. Newhouse, Eric C. Schneider, Bill J. Wright, Alan M. Zaslavsky, and Amy N. Finkelstein, "The Oregon Experiment—Effects of Medicaid on Clinical Outcomes," *New England Journal of Medicine*, Vol. 368, No. 18, 2013, pp. 1713–1722.

Barnett, Jessica C., and Marina S. Vornovitsky, *Current Population Reports, Health Insurance Coverage in the United States: 2015*, Washington, D.C.: United States Census Bureau, P60-257(RV), 2016.

California Department of Insurance, "Provider Network Adequacy," web page, undated. As of July 24, 2017:
http://www.insurance.ca.gov/01-consumers/110-health/10-basics/pna.cfm

CBO—*See* Congressional Budget Office.

Centers for Medicare & Medicaid Services, *Health Insurance Marketplaces 2017 Open Enrollment Period Final Enrollment Report: November 1, 2016–January 31, 2017*, Baltimore, Md., 2017a. As of June 29, 2017:
https://www.cms.gov/Newsroom/MediaReleaseDatabase/Fact-sheets/
2017-Fact-Sheet-items/2017-03-15.html

Centers for Medicare & Medicaid Services, "Medicaid and CHIP Total Enrollment Chart—April 2017," web page, May 2017b. As of June 29, 2017:
https://www.medicaid.gov/medicaid/program-information/
medicaid-and-chip-enrollment-data/report-highlights/total-enrollment/index.html

Chan, S. H., J. F. Burgess, J. A. Clark, and M. F. Mayo-Smith, "Experience of the Veterans Health Administration in Massachusetts After State Health Care Reform," *Military Medicine*, Vol. 179, No. 11, 2014, pp. 1288–1292, https://doi.org/10.7205/MILMED-D-14-00093.

Claxton, Gary, Cynthia Cox, Anthony Damico, Larry Levitt, and Karen Pollitz, "Pre-Existing Conditions and Medical Underwriting in the Individual Insurance Market Prior to the ACA," Menlo Park, Calif.: Kaiser Family Foundation, 2016.

Congressional Budget Office, *Congressional Budget Office Cost Estimate: H.R. 1628 Better Care Reconciliation Act of 2017*, Washington, D.C., 2017a.

Congressional Budget Office, *H.R. 1628 Better Care Reconciliation Act of 2017*, Washington, D.C., 2017b. As of September 6, 2017:
https://www.cbo.gov/system/files/115th-congress-2017-2018/costestimate/
52849-hr1628senate.pdf

Eibner, Christine, Heather Krull, Kristine Brown, Matthew Cefalu, Andrew W. Mulcahy, Michael Pollard, Kanaka Shetty, David M. Adamson, Ernesto F. L. Amaral, Philip Armour, Trinidad Beleche, Olena Bogdan, Jaime L. Hastings, Kandice Kapinos, Amii Kress, Joshua Mendelsohn, Rachel Ross, Carolyn M. Rutter, Robin M. Weinick, Dulani Woods, Susan D. Hosek, and Carrie M. Farmer, *Current and Projected Characteristics and Unique Health Care Needs of the Patient Population Served by the Department of Veterans Affairs*, Santa Monica, Calif.: RAND Corporation, RR-1165/1-VA, 2015. As of June 27, 2017: https://www.rand.org/pubs/research_reports/RR1165z1.html

Eibner, Christine, Jodi Liu, and Sarah Nowak, *The Effects of the American Health Care Act on Health Insurance Coverage and Federal Spending in 2020 and 2026*, Santa Monica, Calif.: RAND Corporation, RR-2003-CMF, 2017. As of July 7, 2017: https://www.rand.org/pubs/research_reports/RR2003.html

Fiedler, Matthew, *Allowing States to Define "Essential Health Benefits" Could Weaken ACA Protections Against Catastrophic Costs for People with Employer Coverage Nationwide*, Washington, D.C.: Brookings Institution, 2017.

Finkelstein, Amy, Sarah Taubman, Bill Wright, Mira Bernstein, Jonathan Gruber, Joseph P. Newhouse, Heidi Allen, Katherine Baicker, and Oregon Health Study Group, "The Oregon Health Insurance Experiment: Evidence from the First Year," *Quarterly Journal of Economics*, Vol. 127, No. 3, 2012, pp. 1057–1106.

Frakt, Austin B., Amresh Hanchate, and Steven D. Pizer, "The Effect of Medicaid Expansions on Demand for Care from the Veterans Health Administration," *Healthcare*, Vol. 3, No. 3, 2015, pp. 123–128.

Frean, Molly, Jonathan Gruber, and Benjamin D. Sommers, "Premium Subsidies, the Mandate, and Medicaid Expansion: Coverage Effects of the Affordable Care Act," *Journal of Health Economics*, Vol. 53, 2017, pp. 72–86.

Gasper, Joseph, Helen Liu, Sharon Kim, and Laurie May, *2015 Survey of Veteran Enrollees' Health and Use of Health Care*, Washington, D.C.: U.S. Department of Veterans Affairs, 2015. As of June 27, 2017: https://www.va.gov/HEALTHPOLICYPLANNING/SoE2015/ 2015_VHA_SoE_Full_Findings_Report.pdf

Haley, Jennifer M., Genevieve M. Kenney, and Jason Gates, *Veterans Saw Broad Coverage Gains Between 2013 and 2015*, Washington, D.C.: Urban Institute, 2017. As of June 27, 2017: http://www.urban.org/research/publication/ veterans-saw-broad-coverage-gains-between-2013-and-2015

Health Affairs, *Health Policy Briefs: Regulation of Health Plan Provider Networks*, July 28, 2016. As of July 24, 2017: http://www.healthaffairs.org/healthpolicybriefs/brief.php?brief_id=160

Holder, Kelly, and David Raglin, *Evaluation of the Revised Veteran Status Question in the 2013 American Community Survey*, Washington, D.C.: U.S. Census Bureau, 2014.

Huang, Grace, Sharon Kim, Joseph Gasper, Yiling Xu, Thomas Bosworth, and Laurie May, *2016 Survey of Veteran Enrollees' Health and Use of Health Care*, Washington, D.C.: U.S. Department of Veterans Affairs, 2017.

Jacobson, Gretchen, Tricia Neuman, and MaryBeth Musumeci, "What Could a Medicaid Per Capita Cap Mean for Low-Income People on Medicare?" Menlo Park, Calif.: Kaiser Family Foundation, 2017. As of June 27, 2017:
http://www.kff.org/medicare/issue-brief/
what-could-a-medicaid-per-capita-cap-mean-for-low-income-people-on-medicare/

Lynch, Victoria, and Genevieve M. Kenney, "Improving the American Community Survey for Studying Health Insurance Reform," *Tenth Conference on Health Survey Research Methods*, Hyattsville, Md.: National Center for Health Statistics, 2011, pp. 87–94. As of August 9, 2017:
http://www.srl.uic.edu/hsrm/hsrm10_proceedings.pdf#page=236

Mann, Cindy, and Allison Orris, "AHCA Would Affect Medicare, Too," *To the Point*, The Commonwealth Fund, 2017. As of August 9, 2017:
http://www.commonwealthfund.org/publications/blog/2017/may/ahca-would-affect-medicare

Ruggles, Steven, Katie Genadek, Ronald Goeken, Josiah Grover, and Matthew Sobek, "Integrated Public Use Microdata Series: Version 6.0 [dataset]," Minneapolis: University of Minnesota, 2015.

Saltzman, Evan, and Christine Eibner, *Donald Trump's Health Care Reform Proposals: Anticipated Effects on Insurance Coverage, Out-of-Pocket Costs, and the Federal Deficit*, The Commonwealth Fund, September 2016.
http://www.commonwealthfund.org/publications/issue-briefs/2016/sep/
trump-presidential-health-care-proposal

Shane, Leo, "Shulkin: New Health Care Bill Could Send More Vets to VA for Care," *Military Times*, May 5, 2017. As of June 27, 2017:
http://www.militarytimes.com/articles/shulkin-health-care-bill-more-vets-va

Shen, Yujing, Ann Hendricks, Fenghua Wang, John Gardner, and Lewis E. Kazis, "The Impact of Private Insurance Coverage on Veterans' Use of VA Care: Insurance and Selection Effects," *Health Services Research*, Vol. 43, No. 1p1, 2008, pp. 267–286. As of August 9, 2017:
http://dx.doi.org/10.1111/j.1475-6773.2007.00743.x

U.S. Congress, 115th Cong., American Health Care Act of 2017, Washington, D.C., H.R. 1628, March 20, 2017. As of September 6, 2017:
https://www.congress.gov/bill/115th-congress/house-bill/1628/summary/00

U.S. Department of Veterans Affairs, "VA Simplifies Access to Health Care and Benefits for Veterans with PTSD," Washington, D.C., July 12, 2010. As of August 9, 2017:
https://www.va.gov/opa/pressrel/pressrelease.cfm?id=1922

U.S. Department of Veterans Affairs, "Combat Veteran Eligibility," February 2015. As of August 9, 2017:
https://www.va.gov/healthbenefits/resources/publications/
IB10-438_combat_veteran_eligibility.pdf

U.S. Department of Veterans Affairs, "Diabetes Mellitus Type 2 and Agent Orange," last updated May 4, 2016a. As of July 24, 2017:
https://www.publichealth.va.gov/exposures/agentorange/conditions/diabetes.asp

U.S. Department of Veterans Affairs, "Where Do I Get the Care I Need?" last updated July 12, 2016b. As of July 24, 2017:
https://www.va.gov/health/findcare.asp

U.S. Department of Veterans Affairs, *Medical Programs and Information Technology Programs: Congressional Submission—FY 2018 Funding and FY 2019 Advance Appropriations*, Vol. II, 2017a. As of June 27, 2017:
https://www.va.gov/budget/docs/summary/
fy2018VAbudgetVolumeIImedicalProgramsAndInformationTechnology.pdf

U.S. Department of Veterans Affairs, "Claims Backlog," last updated August 28, 2017b. As of September 6, 2017:
https://www.benefits.va.gov/reports/mmwr_va_claims_backlog.asp

U.S. Department of Veterans Affairs National Center for Veterans Analysis and Statistics, "National Center for Veterans Analysis and Statistics: State/Territories Summary Reports," last updated December 6, 2016. As of June 27, 2017:
https://www.va.gov/vetdata/stateSummaries.asp

U.S. Department of Veterans Affairs National Center for Veterans Analysis and Statistics, "Veteran Population," last updated July 19, 2017. As of August 28, 2017:
https://www.va.gov/vetdata/veteran_population.asp

VA—*See* U.S. Department of Veterans Affairs.

Veterans Access, Choice, and Accountability Act of 2014, Public Law 113-146.

Wong, E. S., M. L. Maciejewski, P. L. Hebert, C. L. Bryson, and C. Liu, "Massachusetts Health Reform and Veterans Affairs Health System Enrollment," *American Journal of Managed Care*, Vol. 20, No. 8, 2014, pp. 629–636.

Yoon, Jean, Megan E. Vanneman, Sharon K. Dally, Amal N. Trivedi, and Ciaran S. Phibbs, "Use of Veterans Affairs and Medicaid Services for Dually Enrolled Veterans," *Health Services Research*, June 13, 2017. As of August 9, 2017:
http://onlinelibrary.wiley.com/doi/10.1111/1475-6773.12727/full